How to use this book

If you are suffering from chronic pain, there are two reasons to keep a log of what you are feeling:

1) By focusing on how your pain develops, you may notice patterns. This can help you to manage your condition.

2) When you meet your doctor they want a general picture of your condition, but your description can be skewed by how you are feeling at the time. If you keep a log, you'll be able to give them a clearer picture of your condition.

A visual log is quicker and easier to use than a written one. When you get up in the morning, and before going to bed at night, Use the pictures to circle the parts of your body where there is pain. Then, inside each circle, put a number from 1 to 9 to describe your pain, where 1 is very slight and 9 is extreme. You can make a note of anything else that you think is relevant; did a particular activity that day trigger some pain, for example?

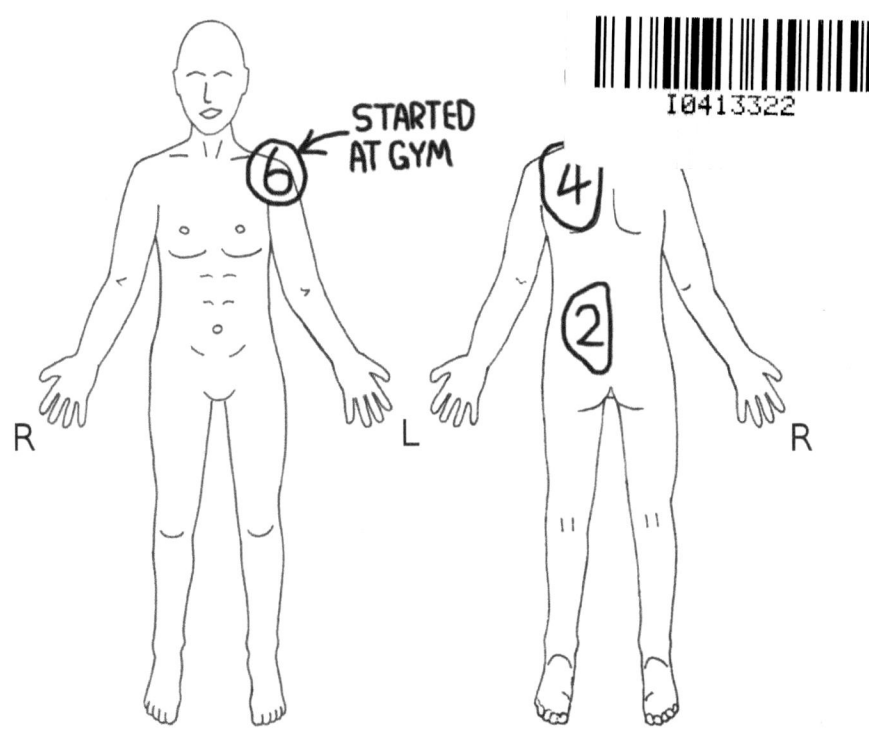

Of course, you can find your own best way to use this book. Any comments and suggestions are welcome: simbamford@gmail.com

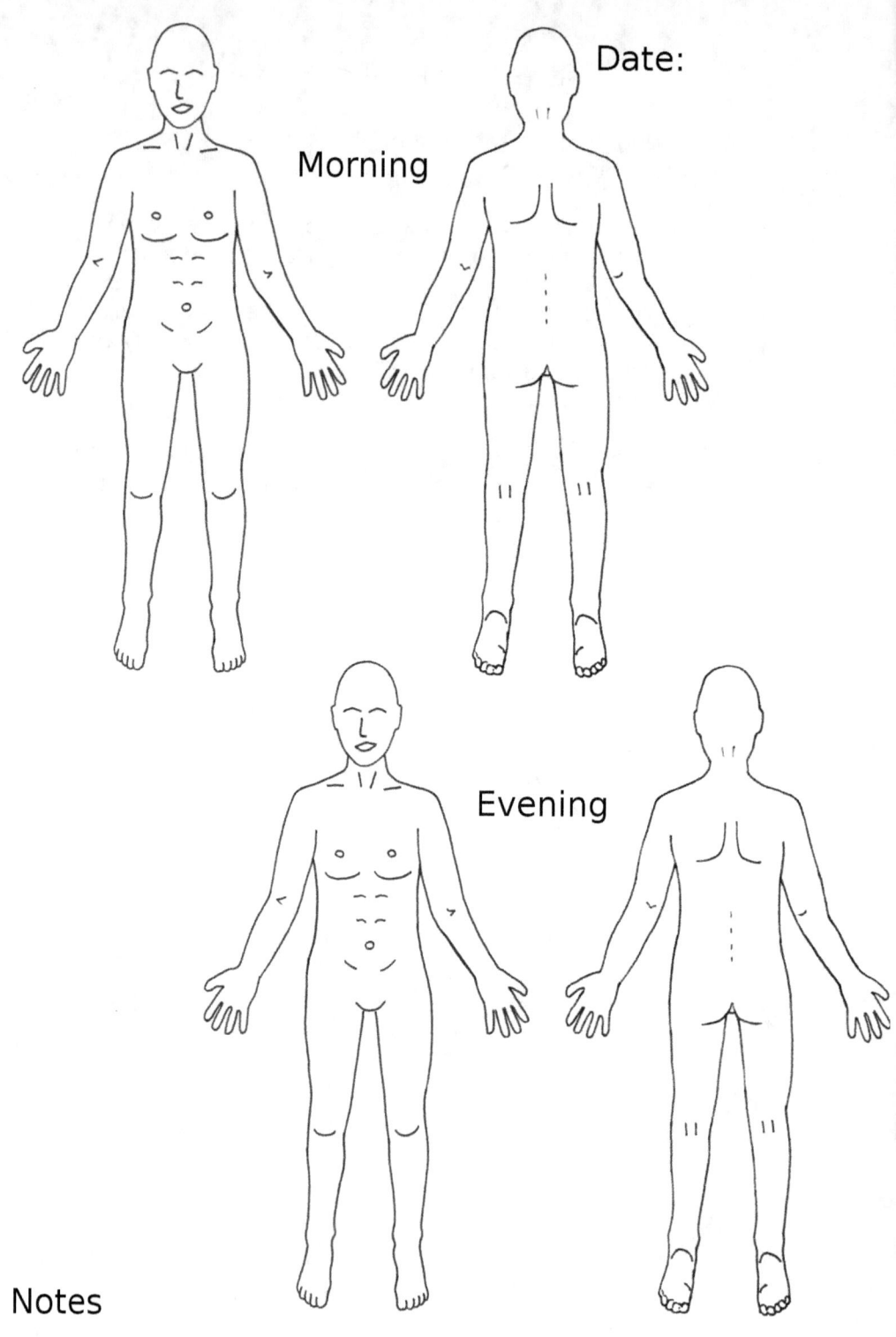

Morning

Date:

Evening

Notes

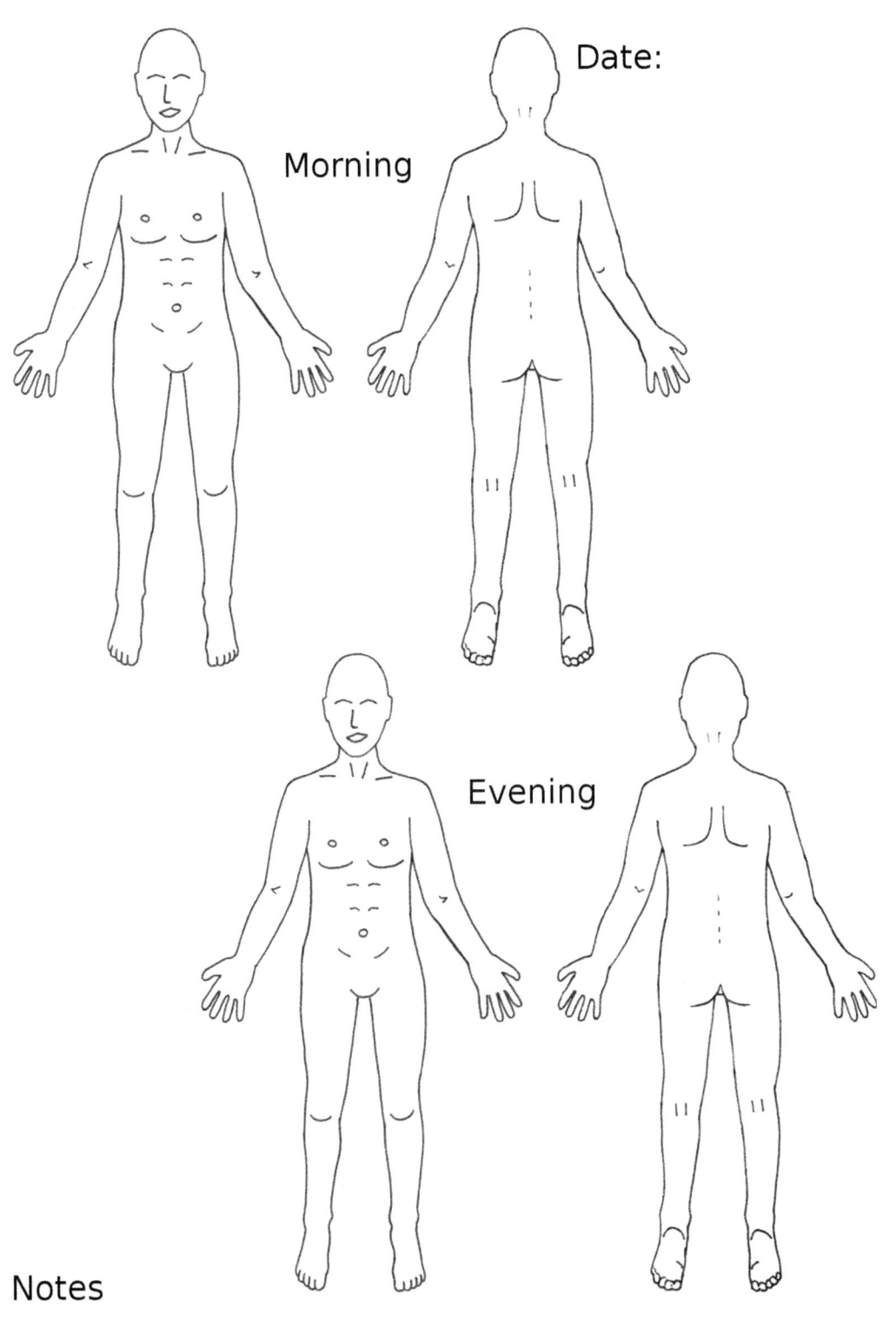

Date:

Morning

Evening

Notes

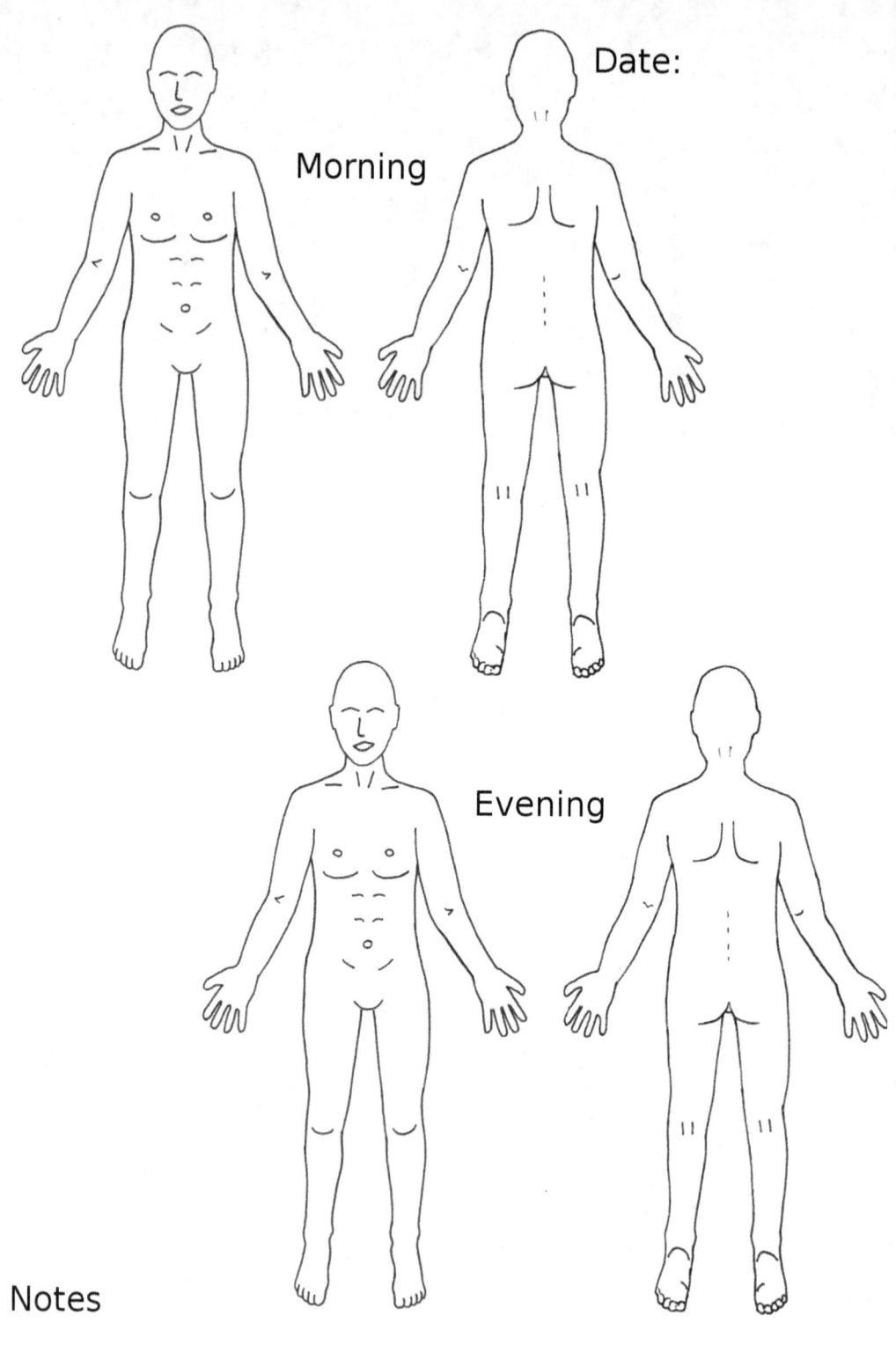

Date:

Morning

Evening

Notes

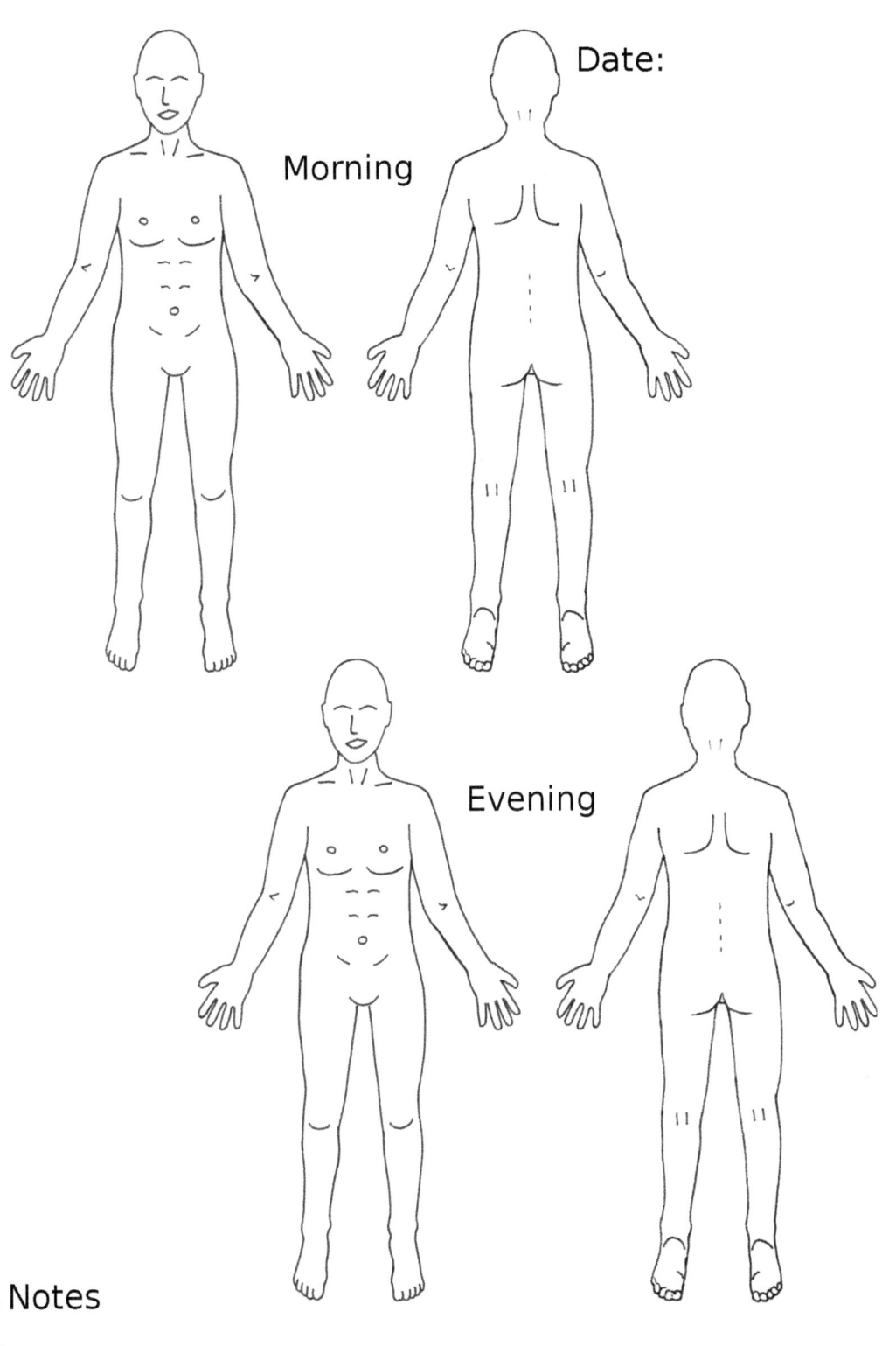

Date:

Morning

Evening

Notes

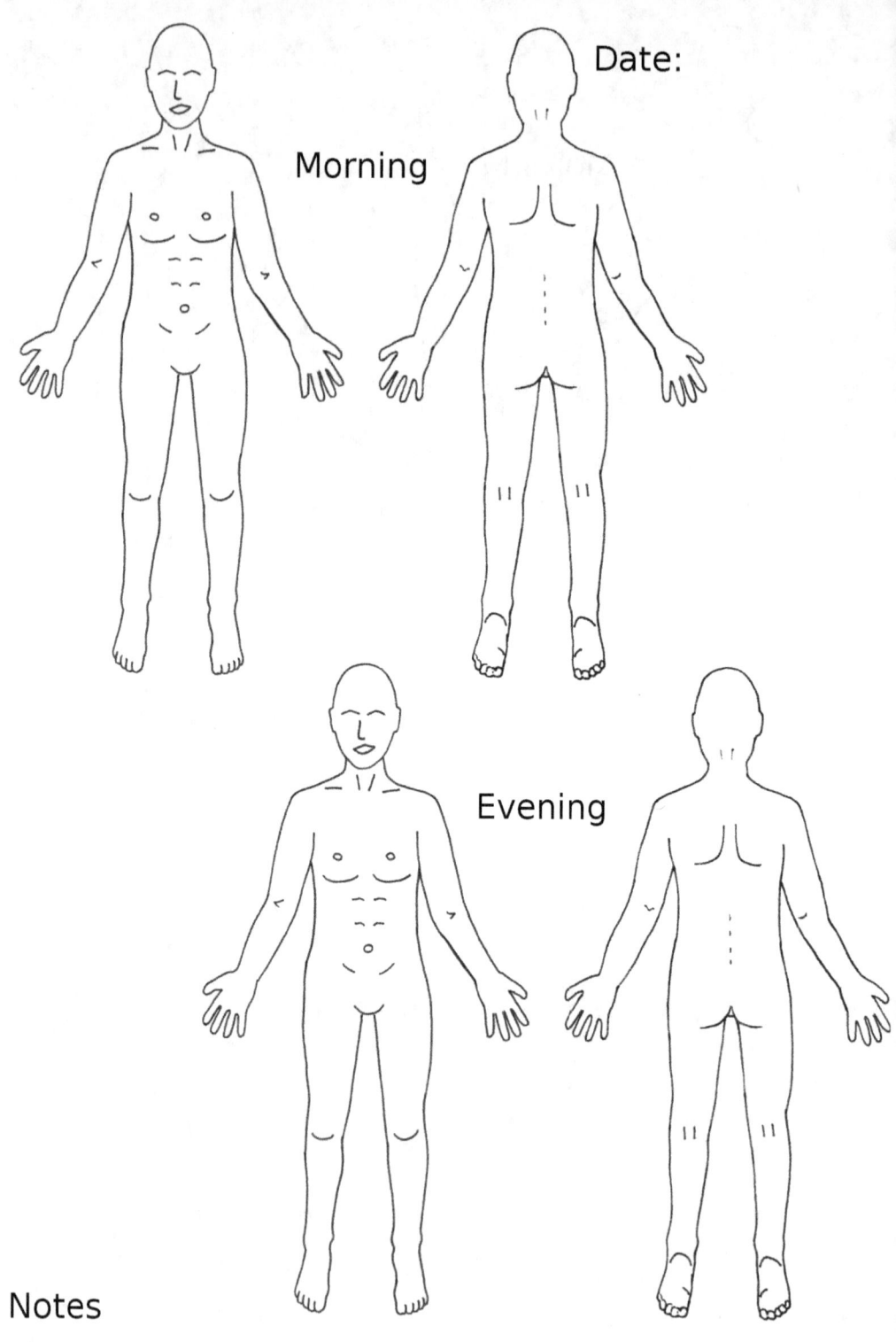

Date:

Morning

Evening

Notes

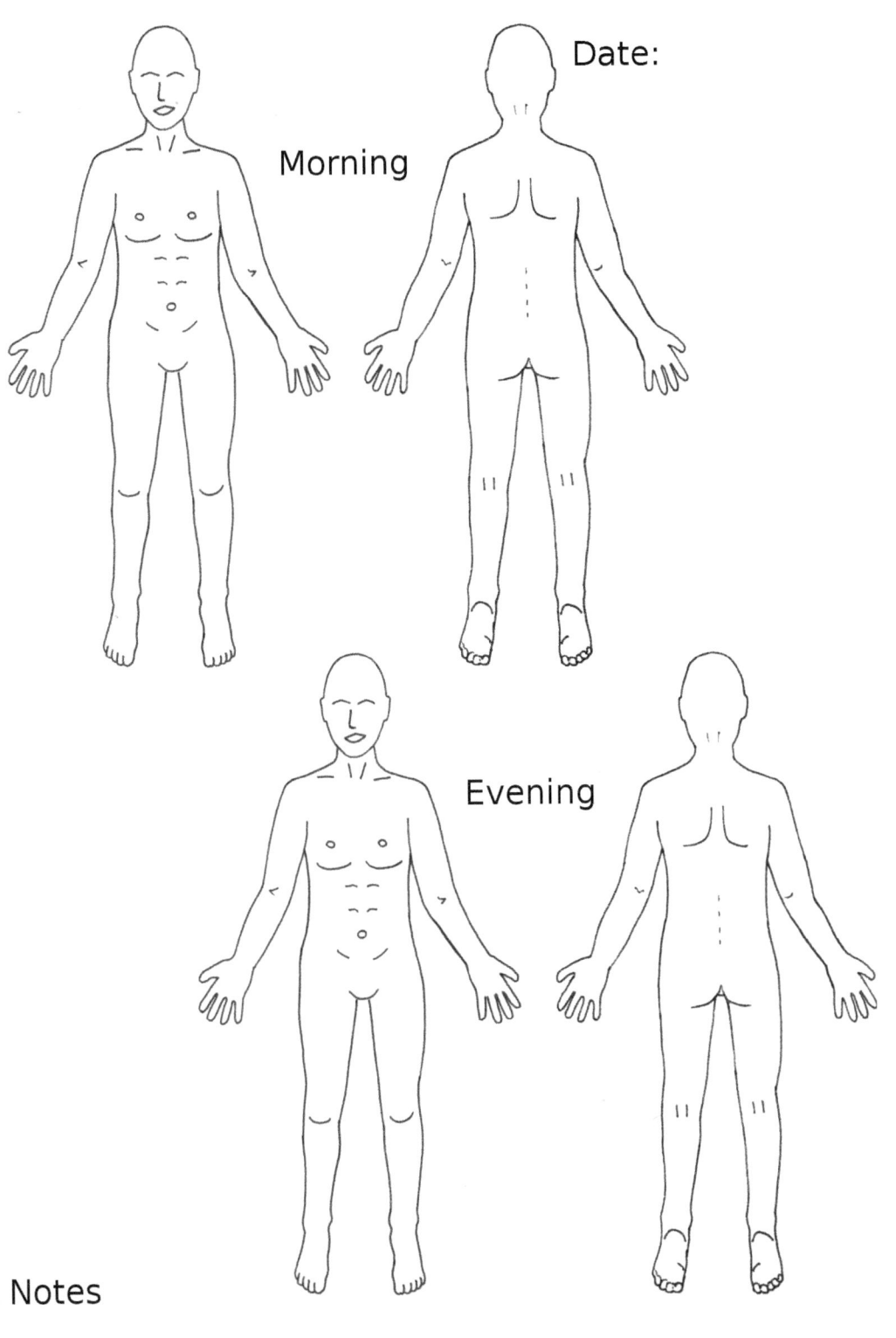

Morning

Date:

Evening

Notes

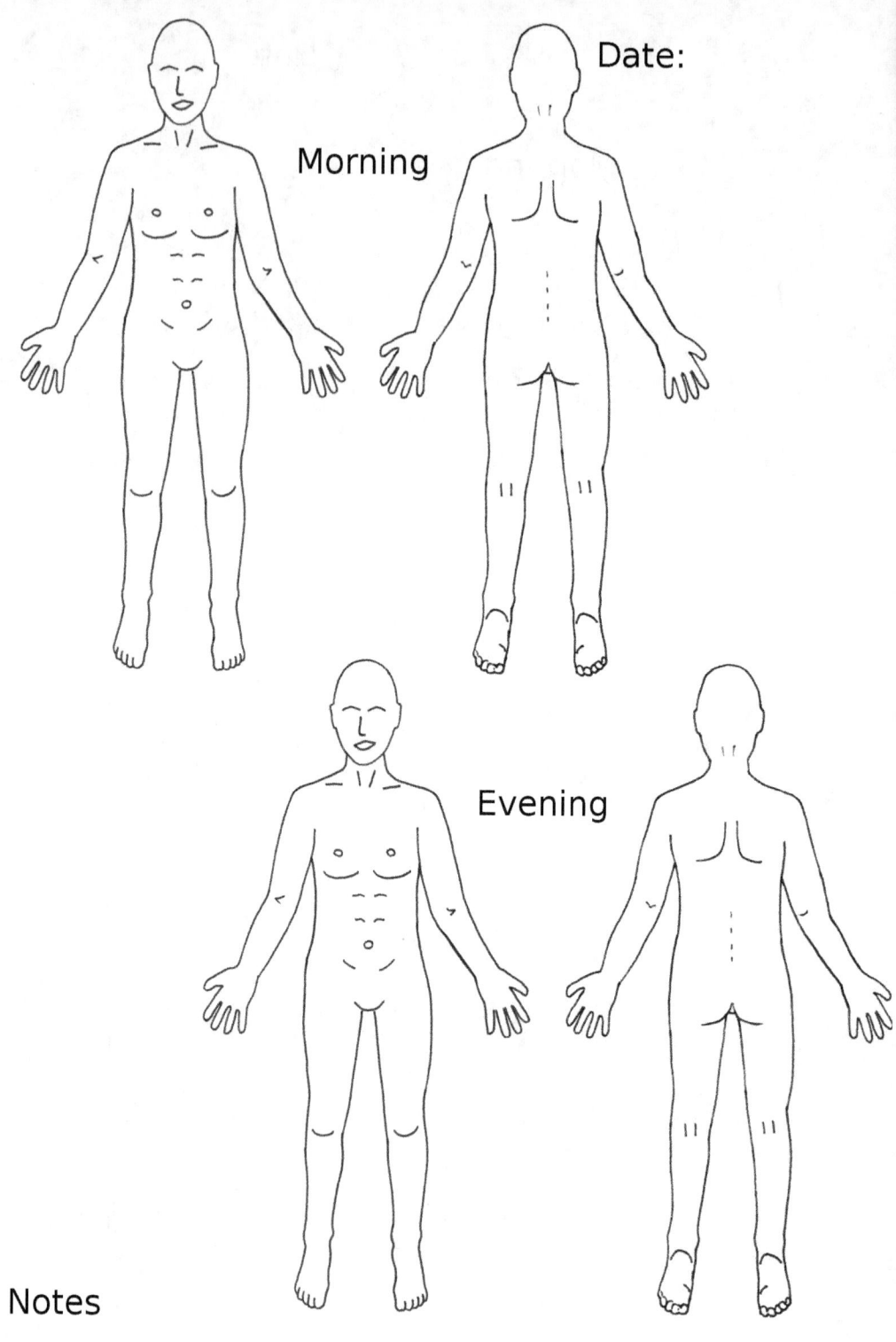

Morning

Date:

Evening

Notes

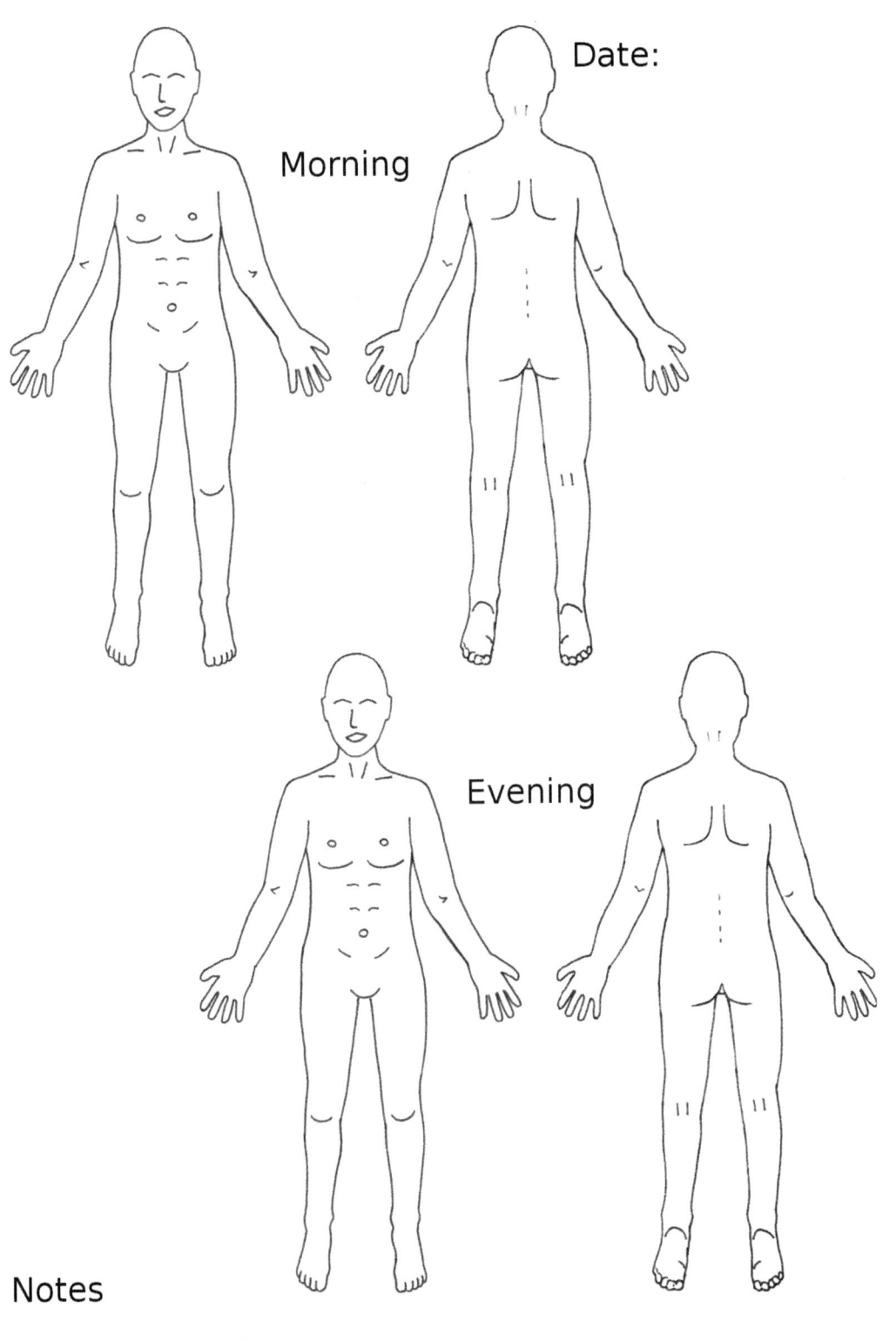

Morning

Date:

Evening

Notes

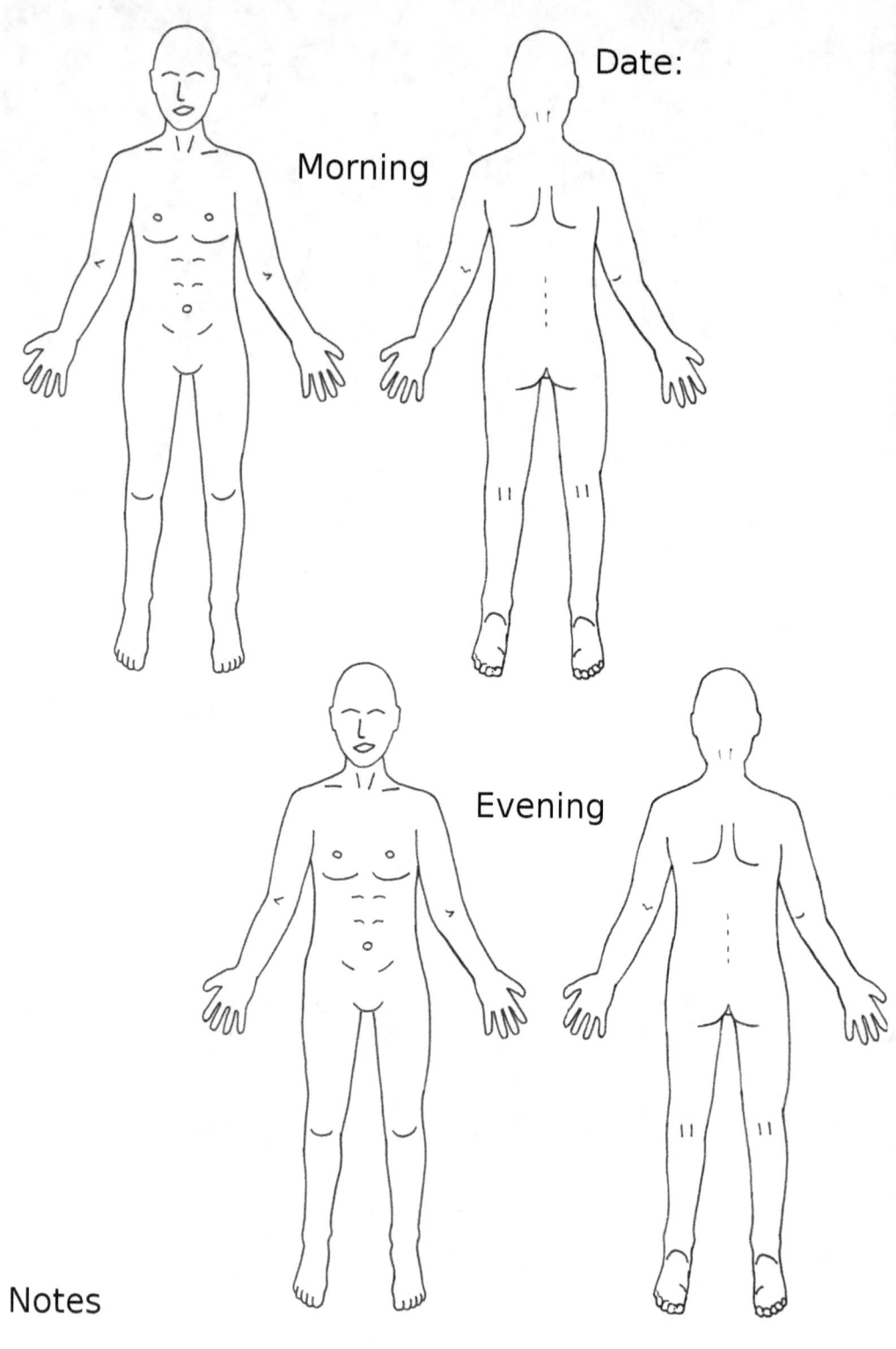

Morning

Date:

Evening

Notes

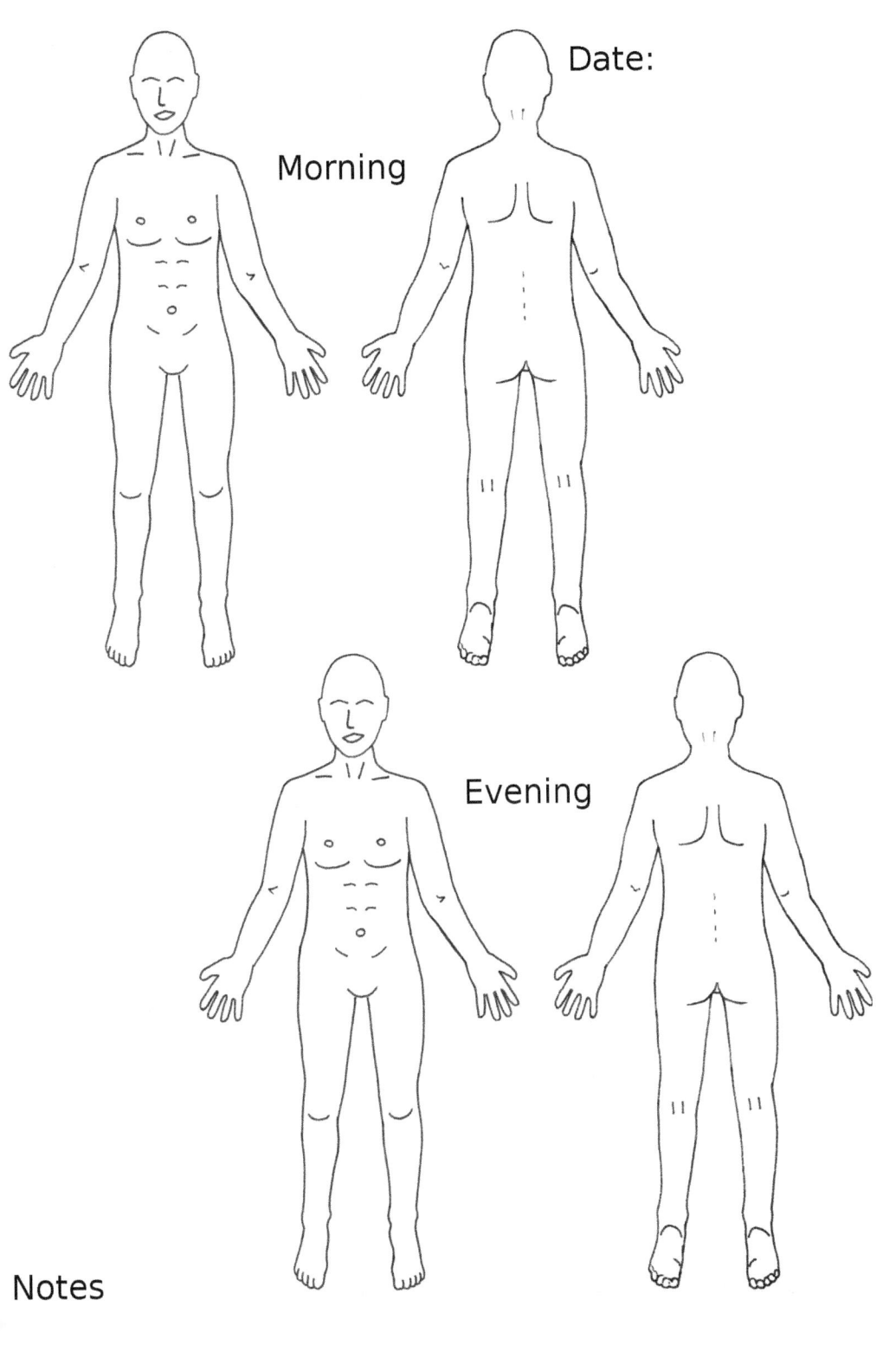

Date:

Morning

Evening

Notes

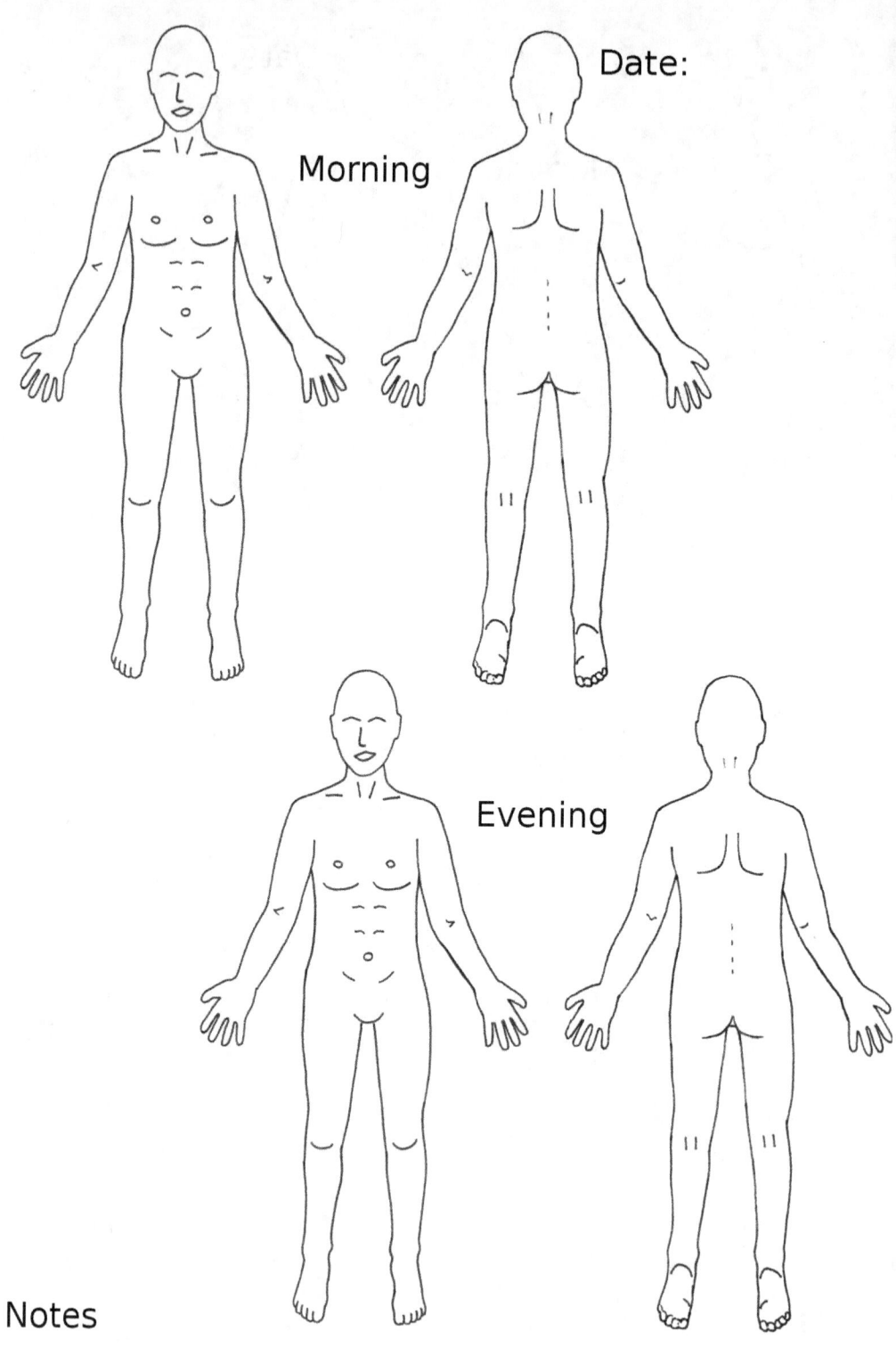

Date:

Morning

Evening

Notes

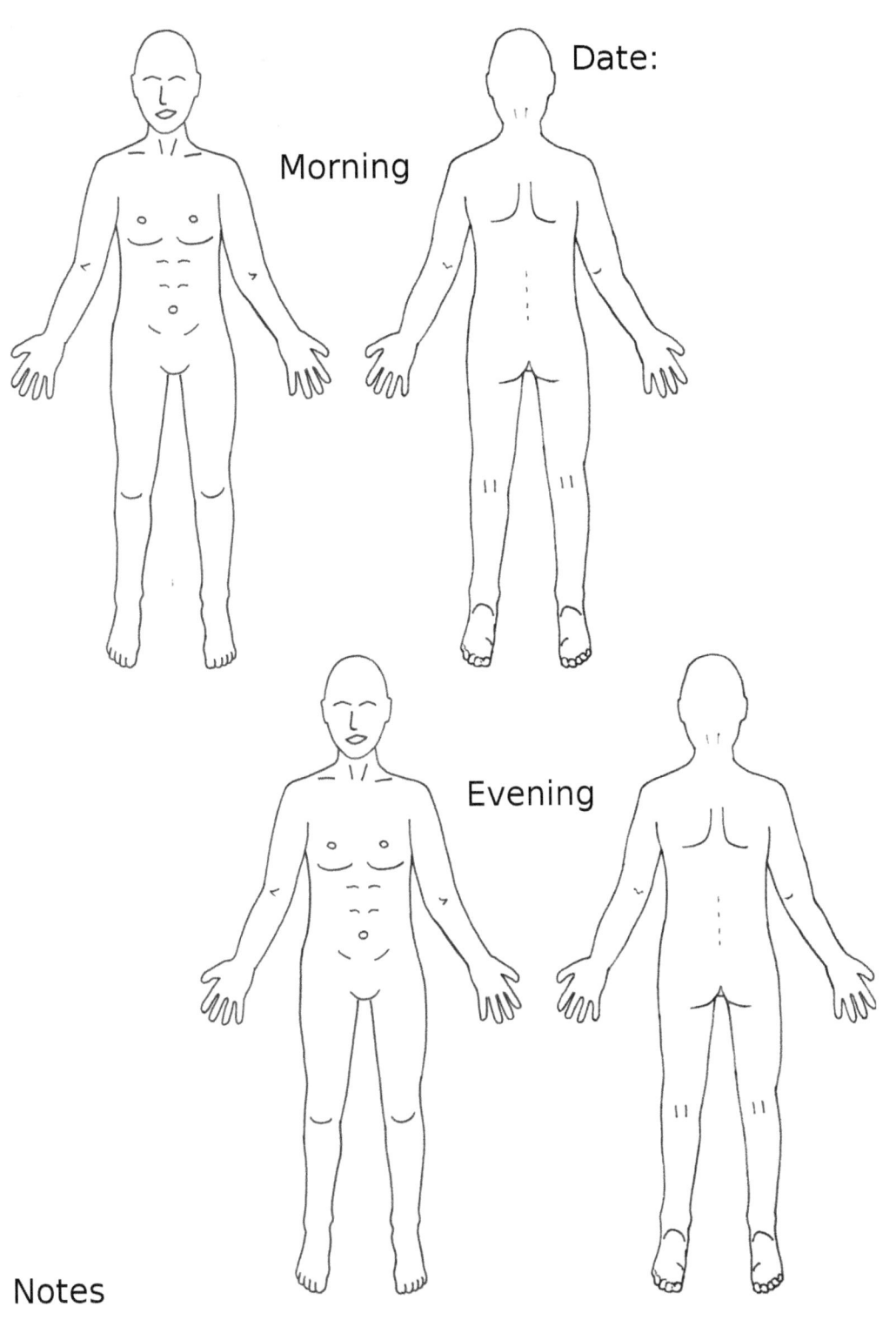

Date:

Morning

Evening

Notes

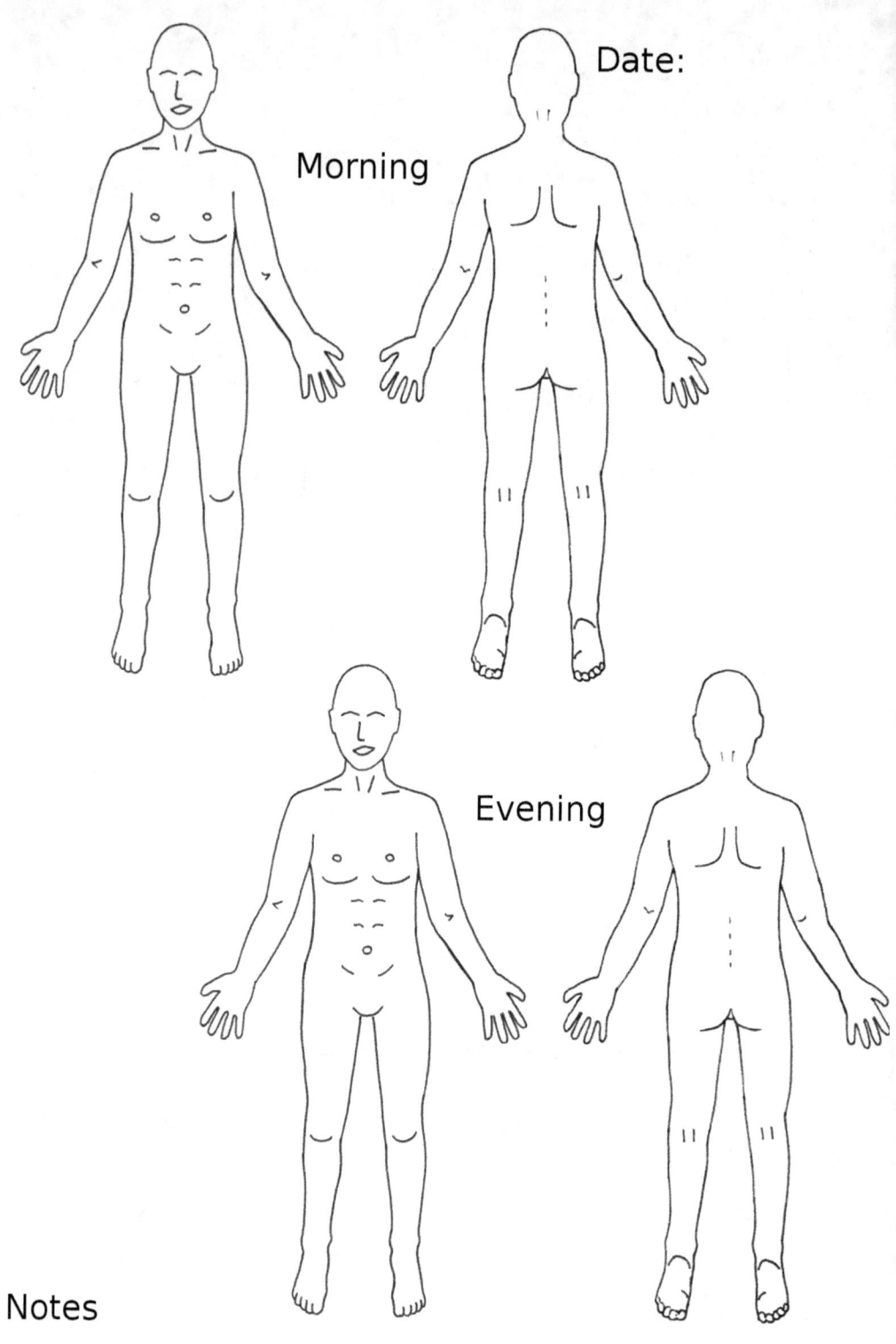

Morning

Date:

Evening

Notes

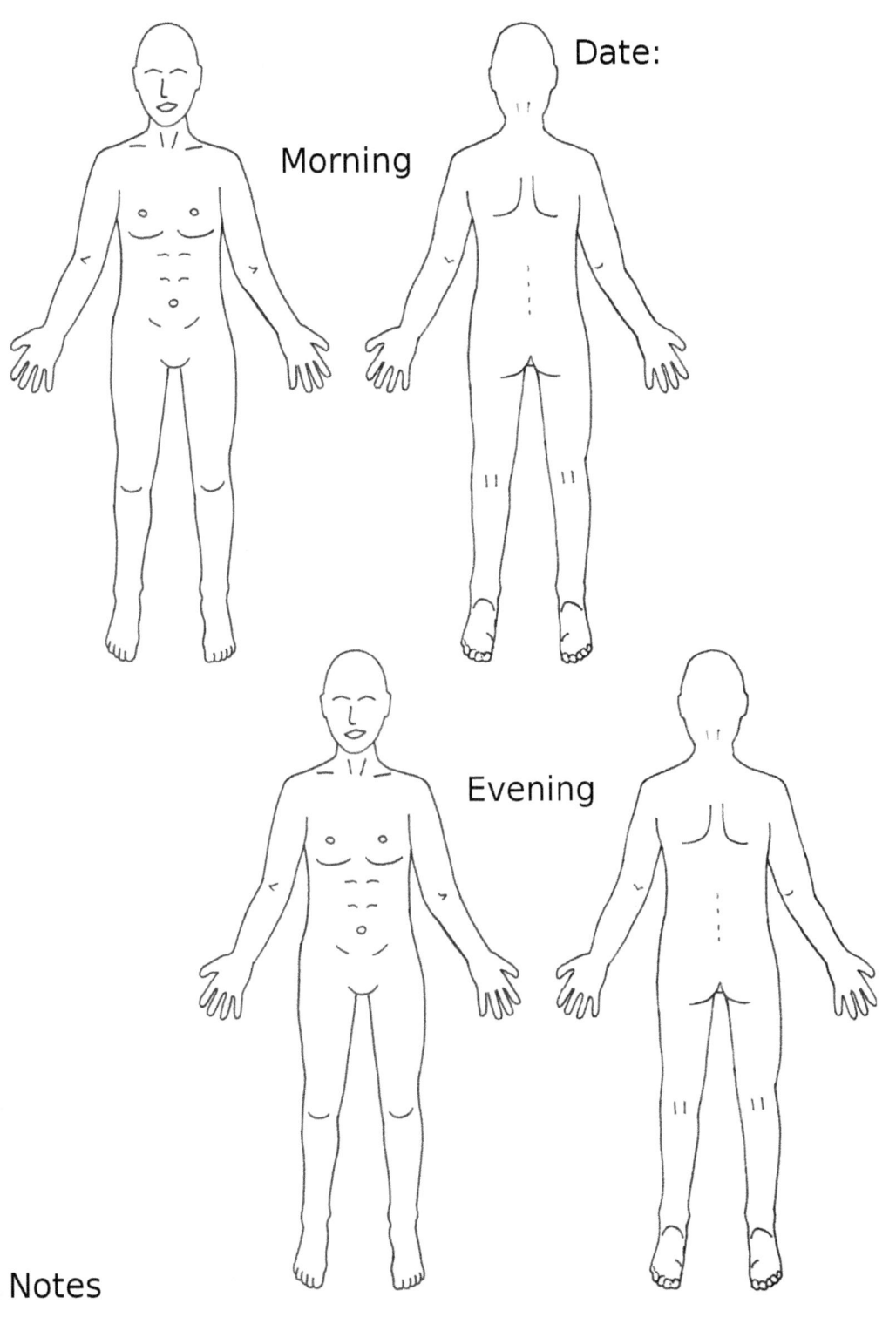

Morning

Date:

Evening

Notes

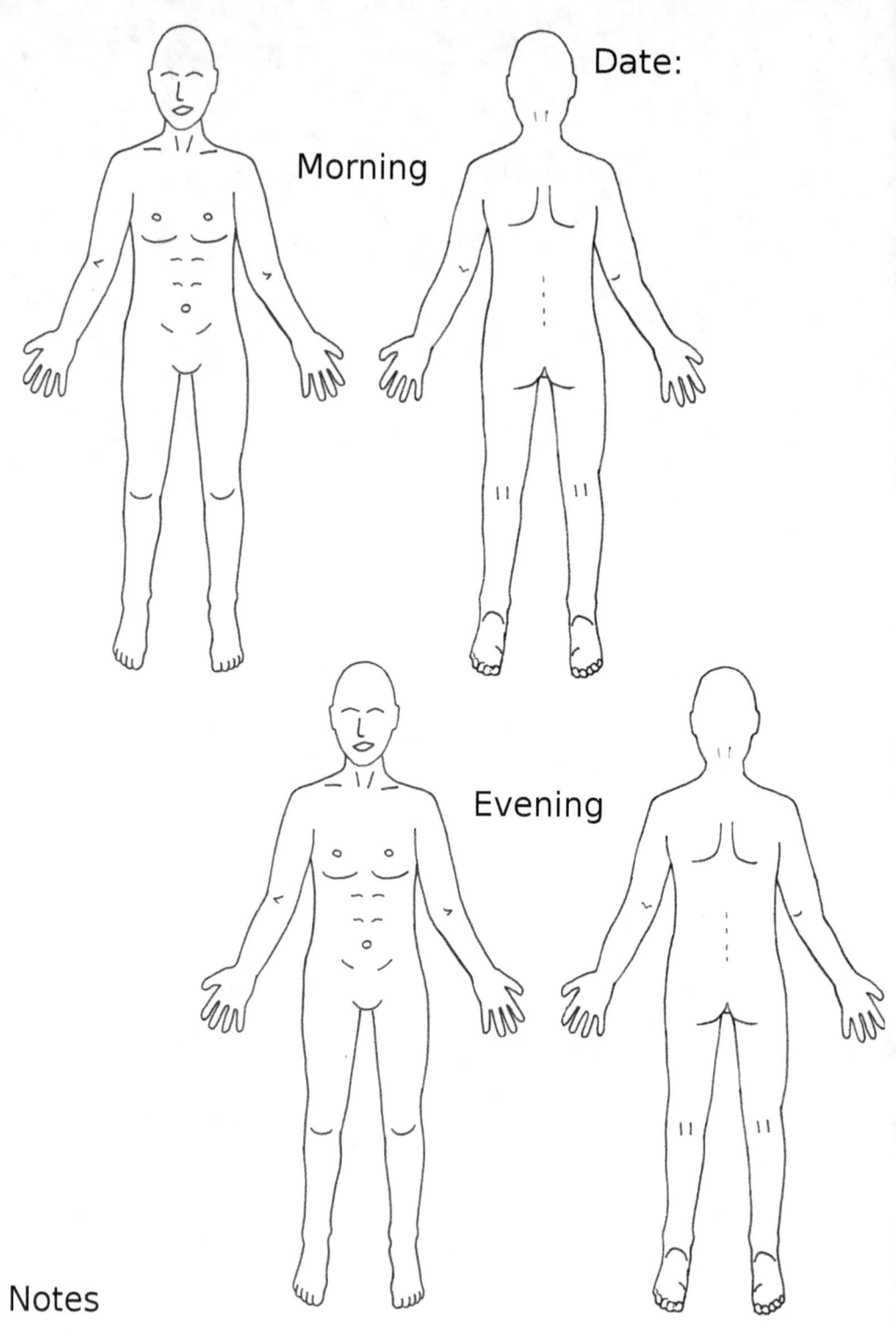

Date:

Morning

Evening

Notes

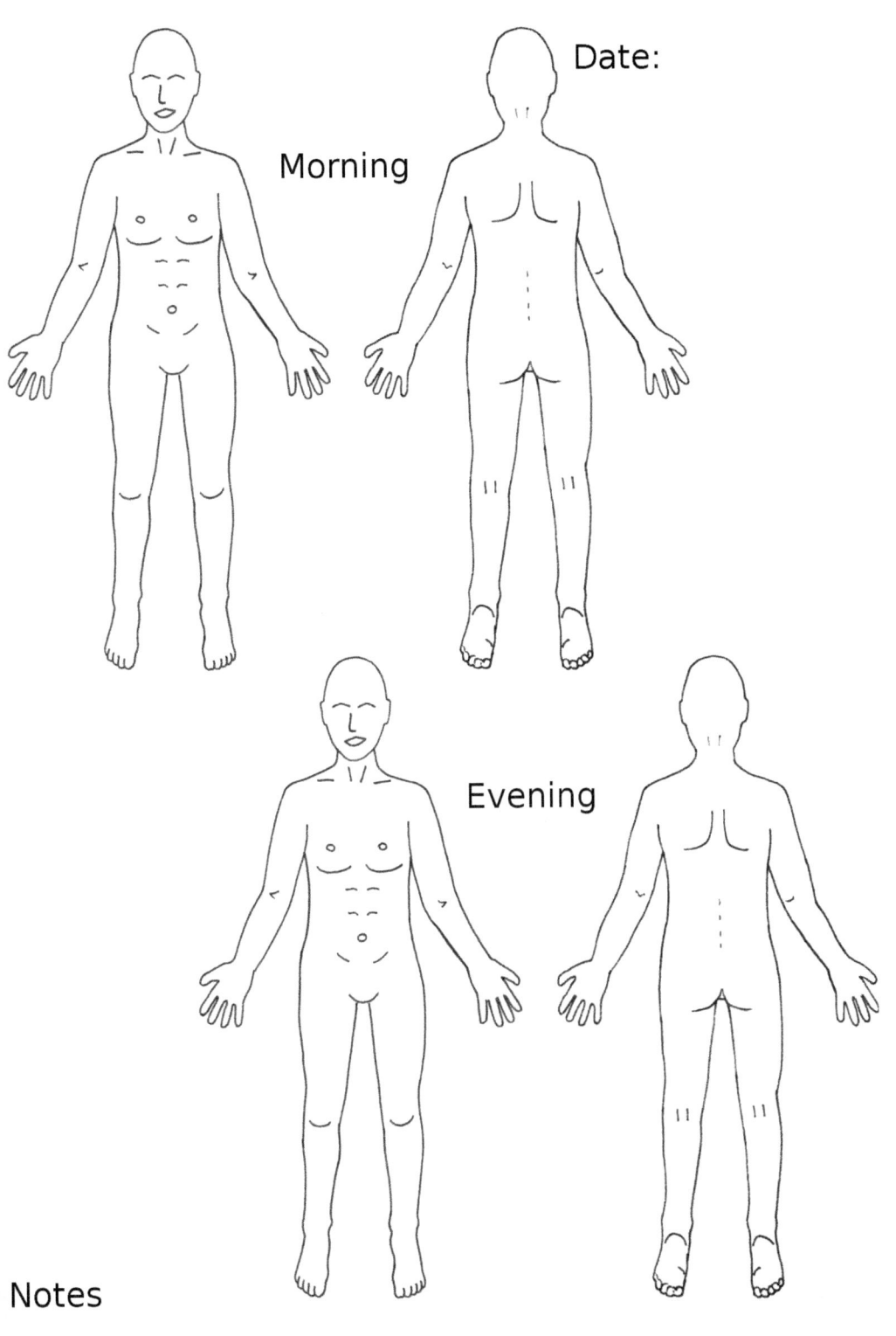

Date:

Morning

Evening

Notes

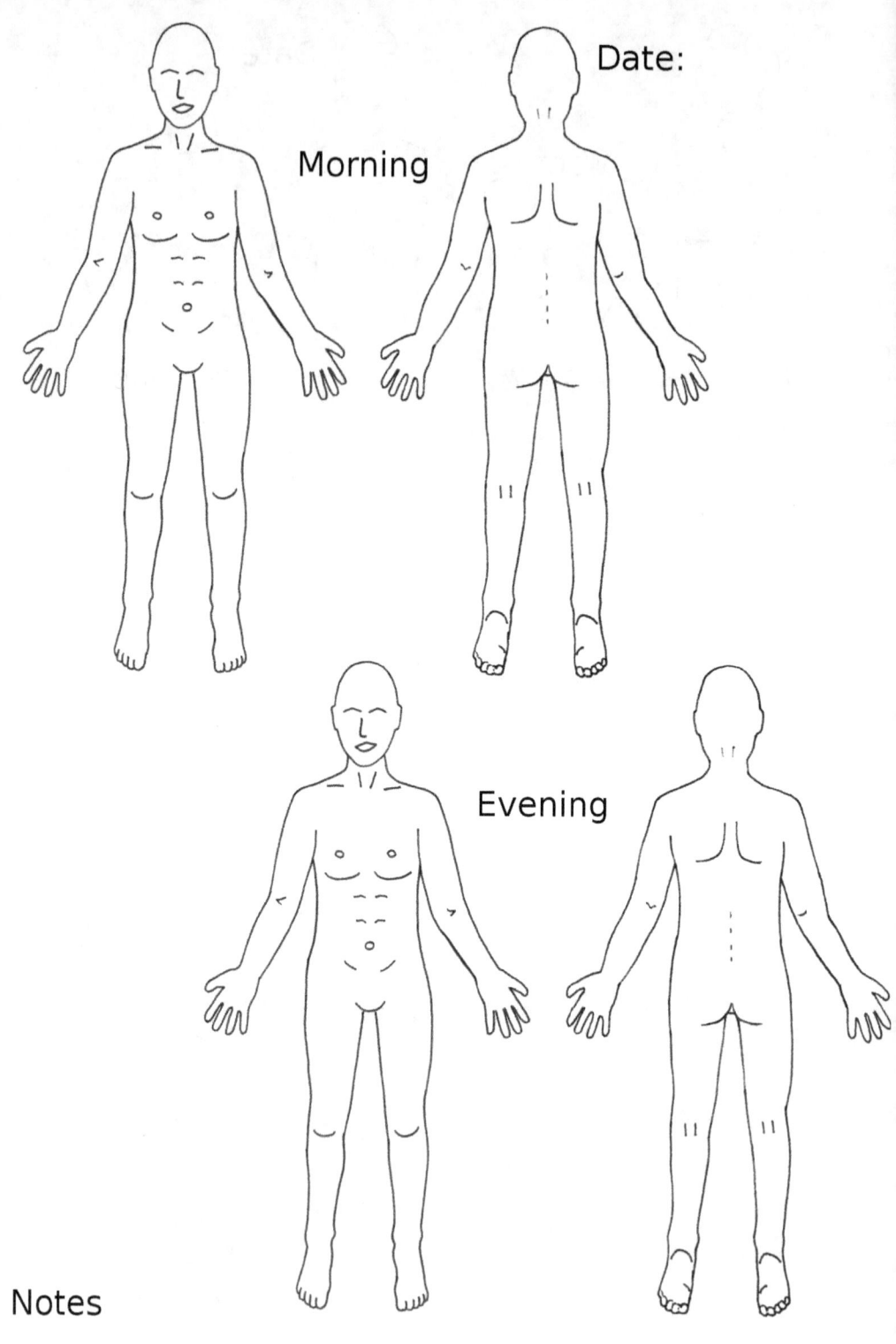

Morning

Date:

Evening

Notes

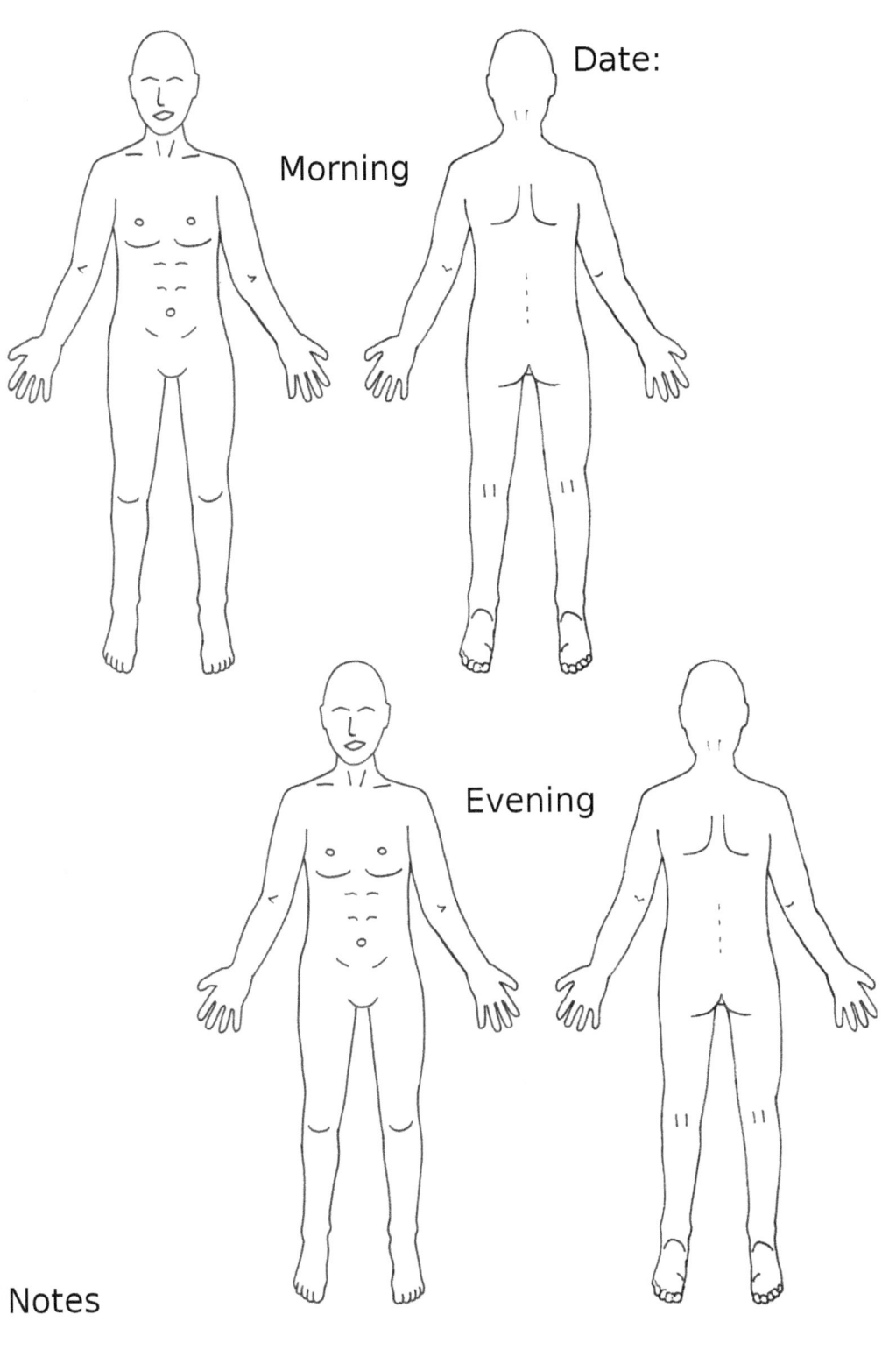

Date:

Morning

Evening

Notes

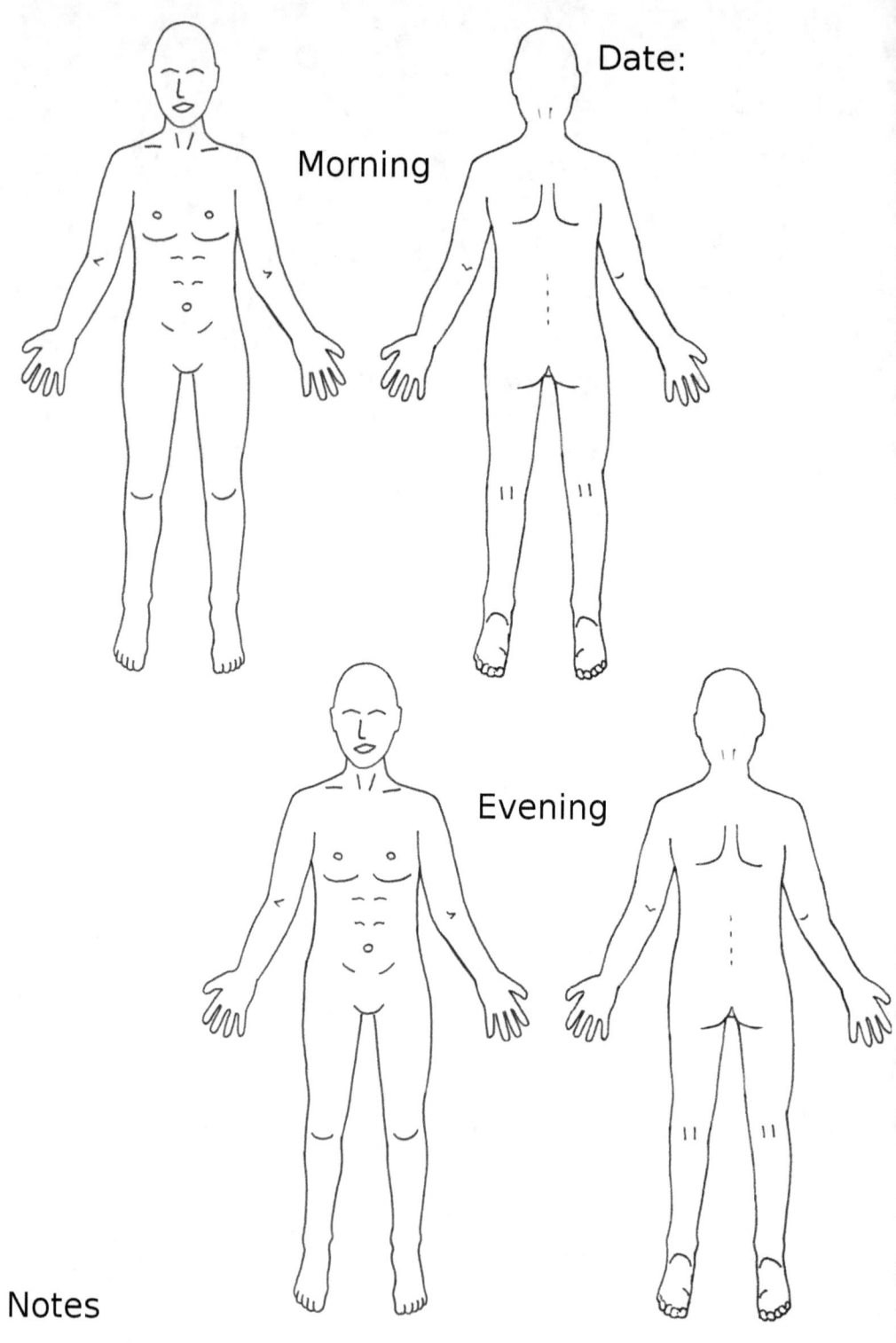

Date:

Morning

Evening

Notes

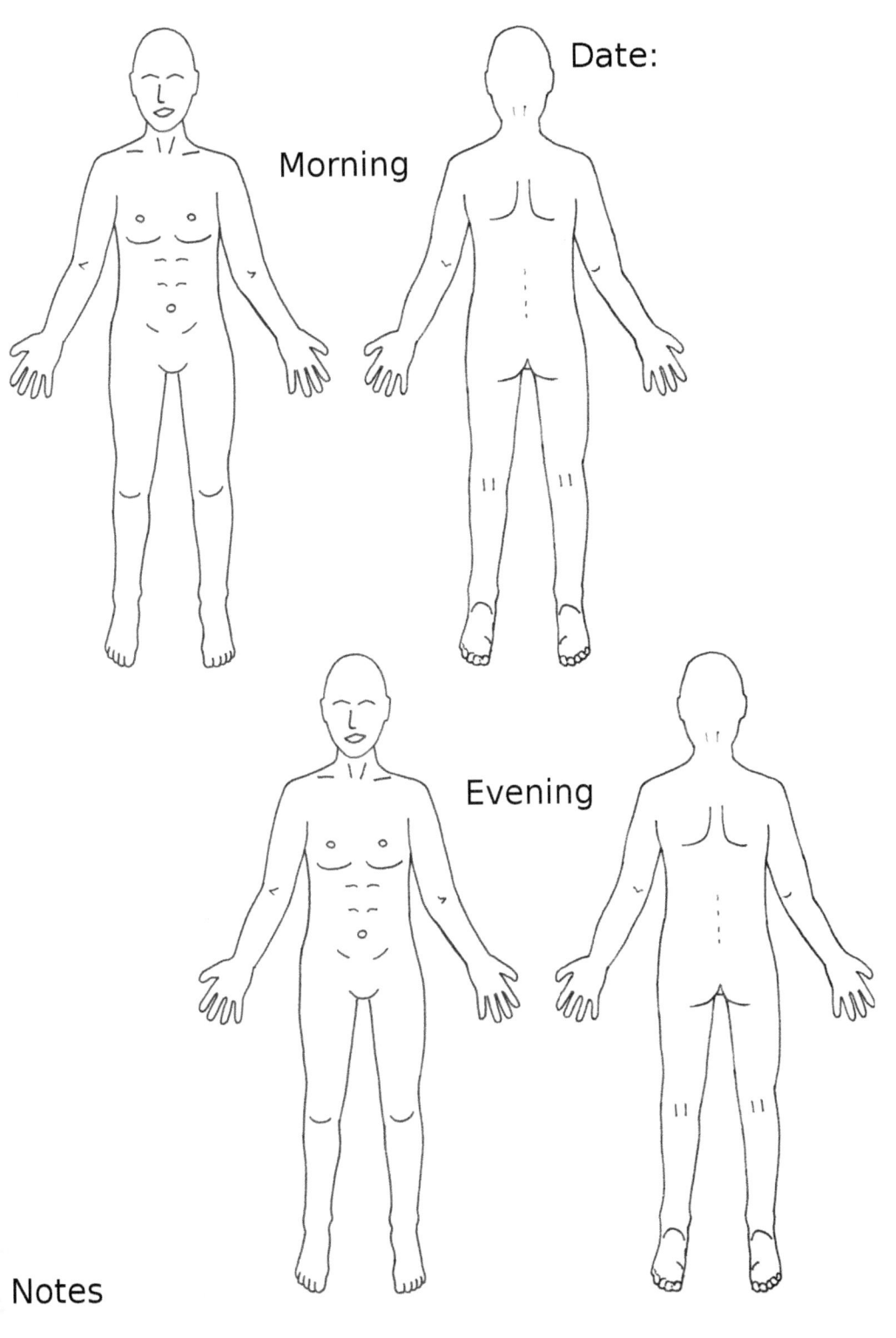

Morning

Date:

Evening

Notes

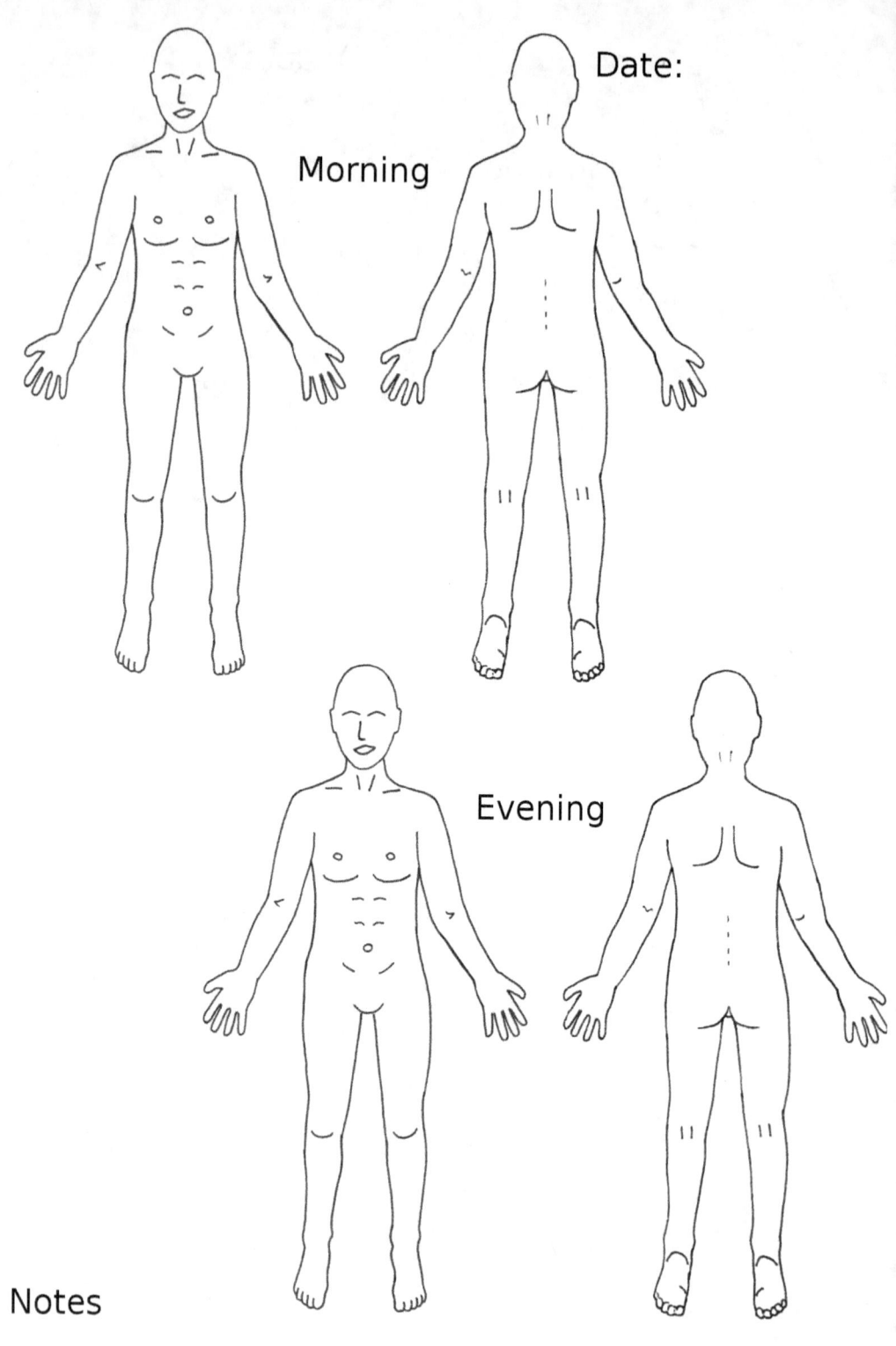

Morning

Date:

Evening

Notes

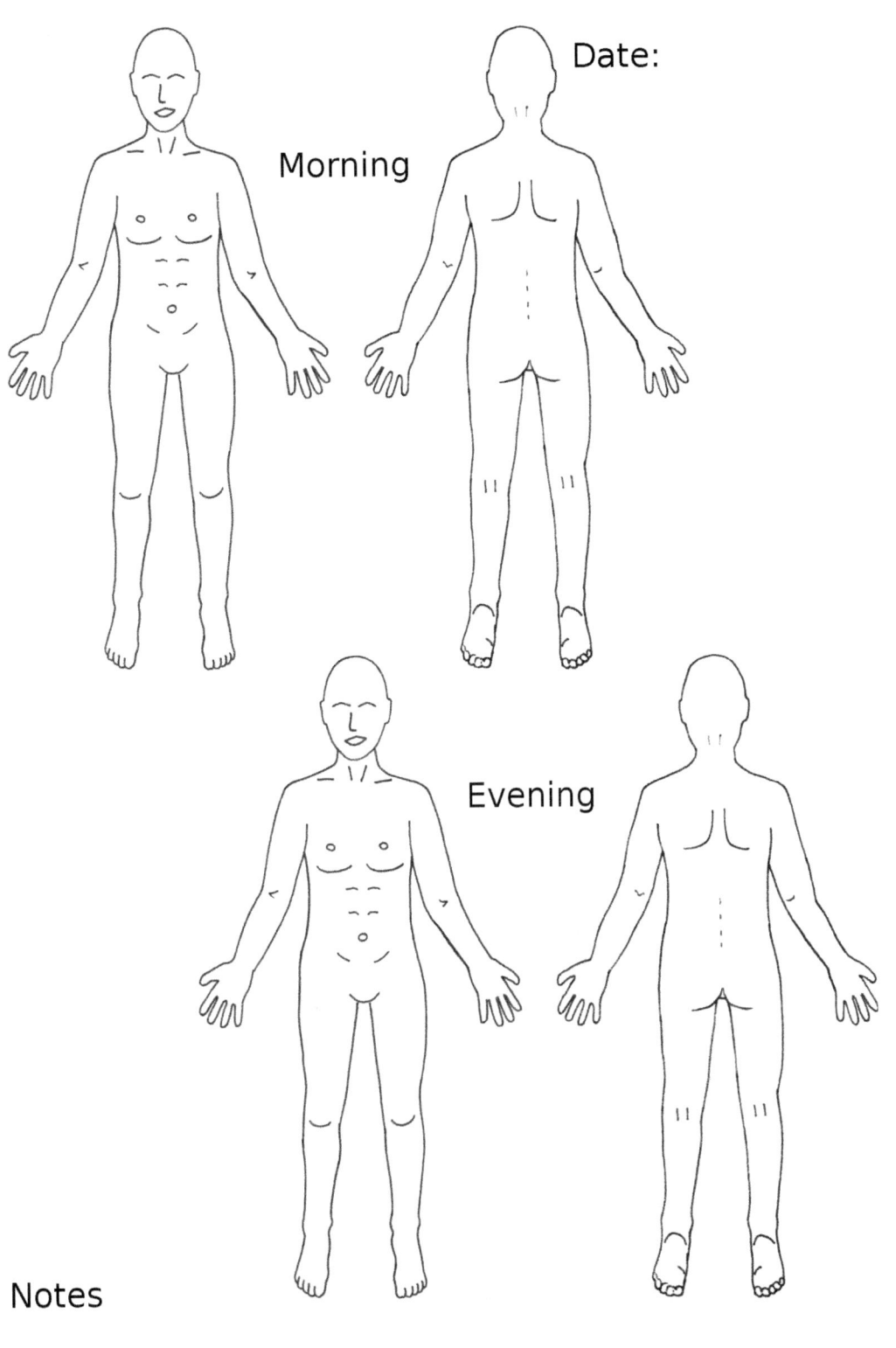

Date:

Morning

Evening

Notes

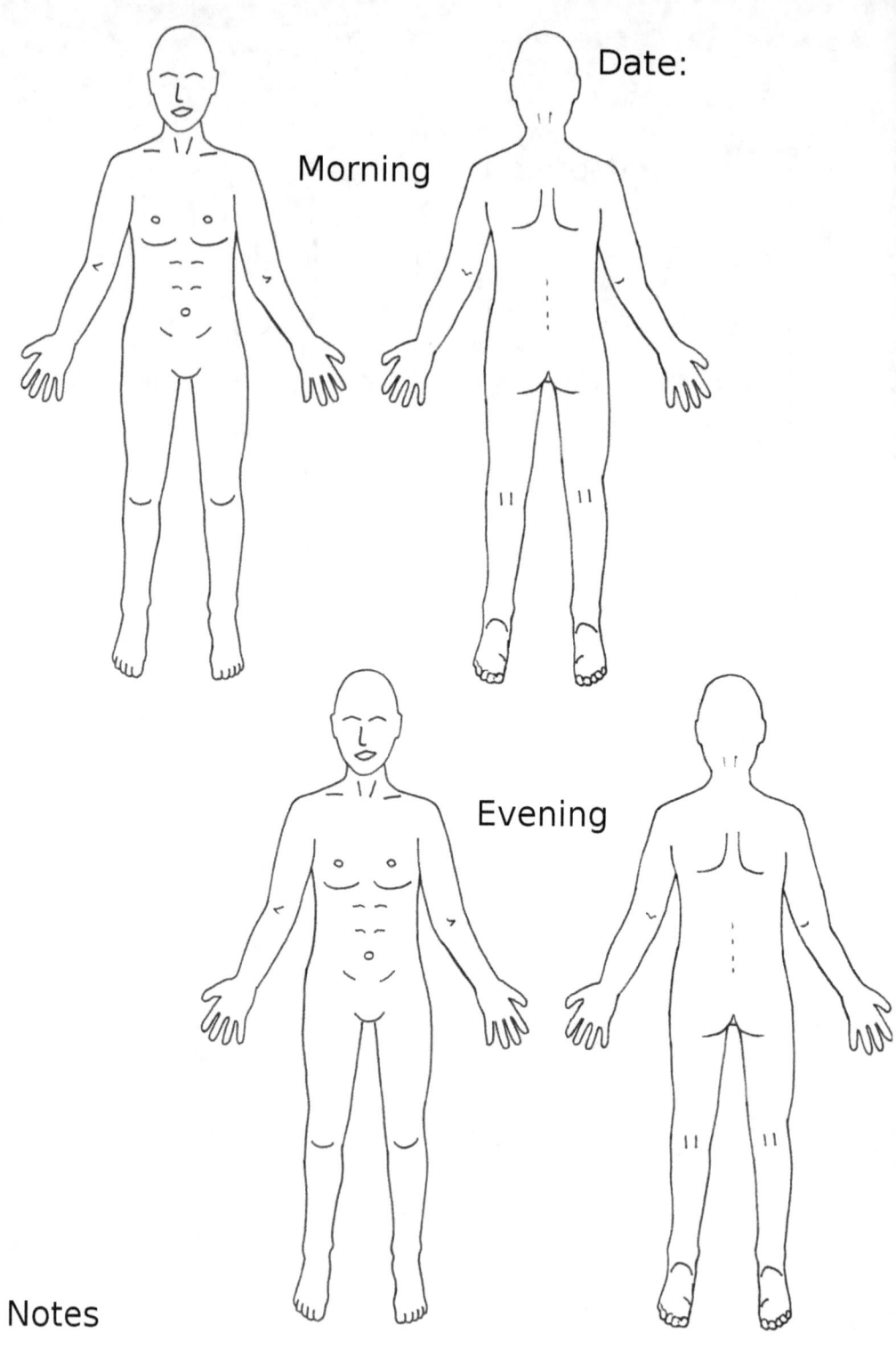

Date:

Morning

Evening

Notes

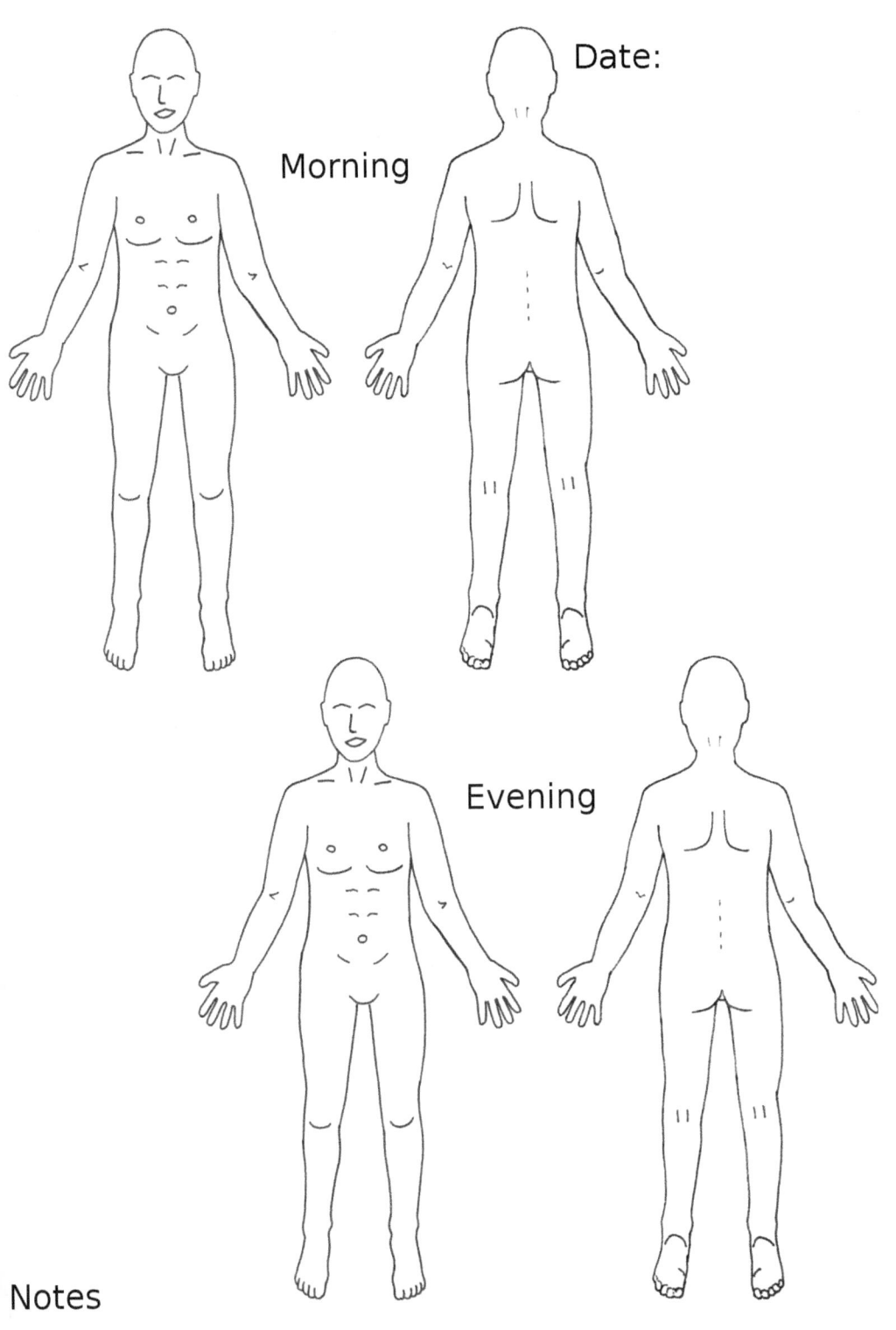

Morning

Date:

Evening

Notes

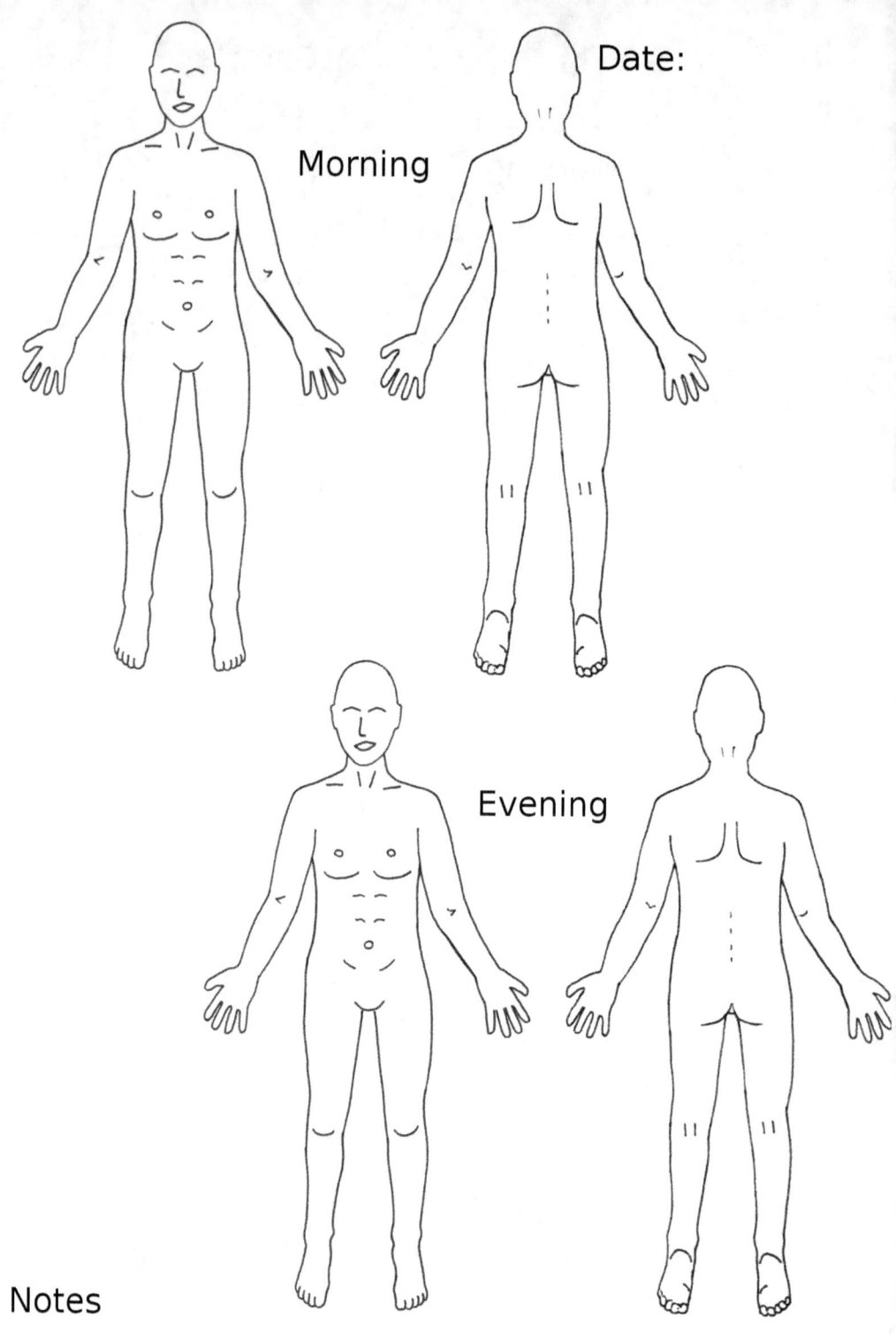

Date:

Morning

Evening

Notes

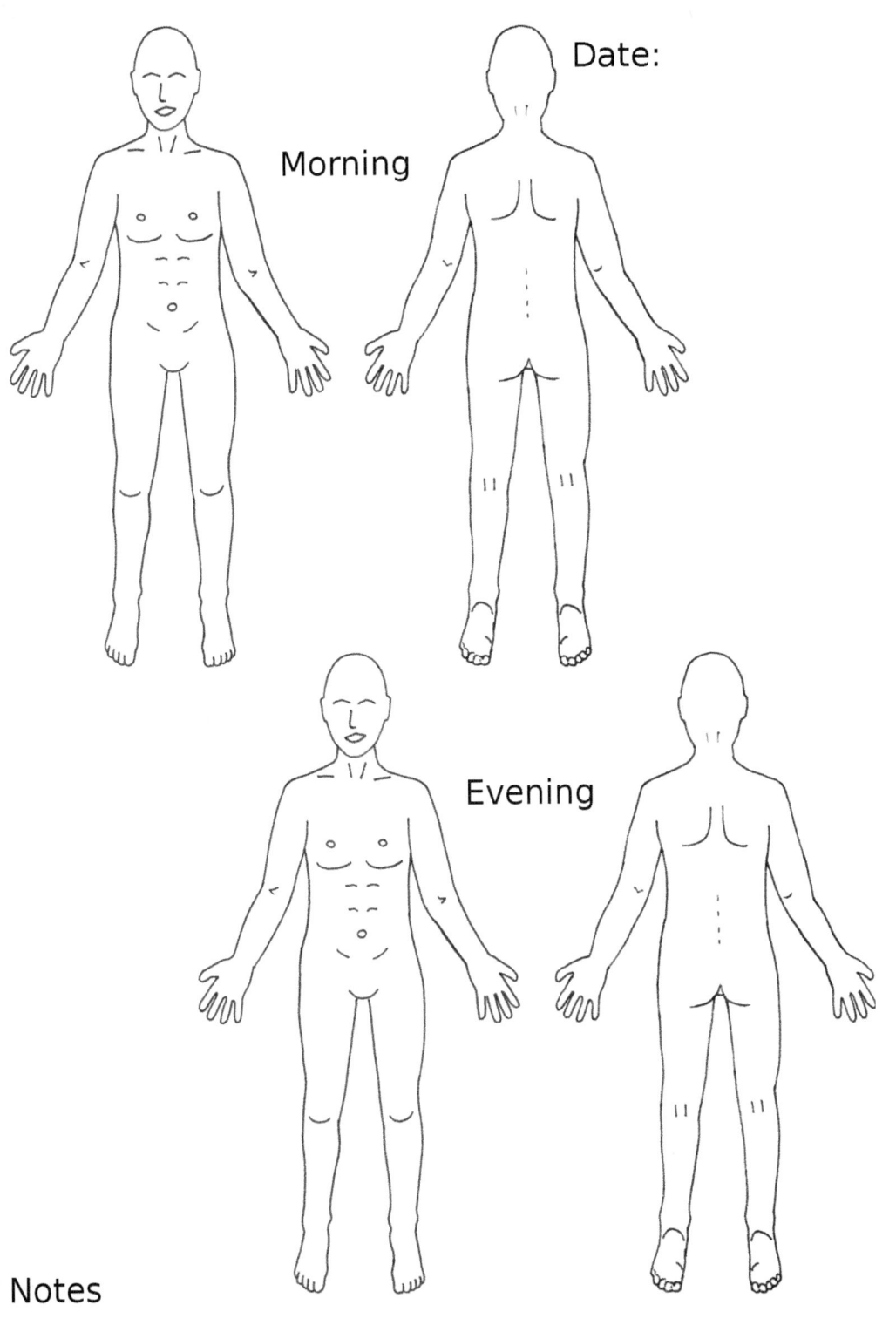

Date:

Morning

Evening

Notes

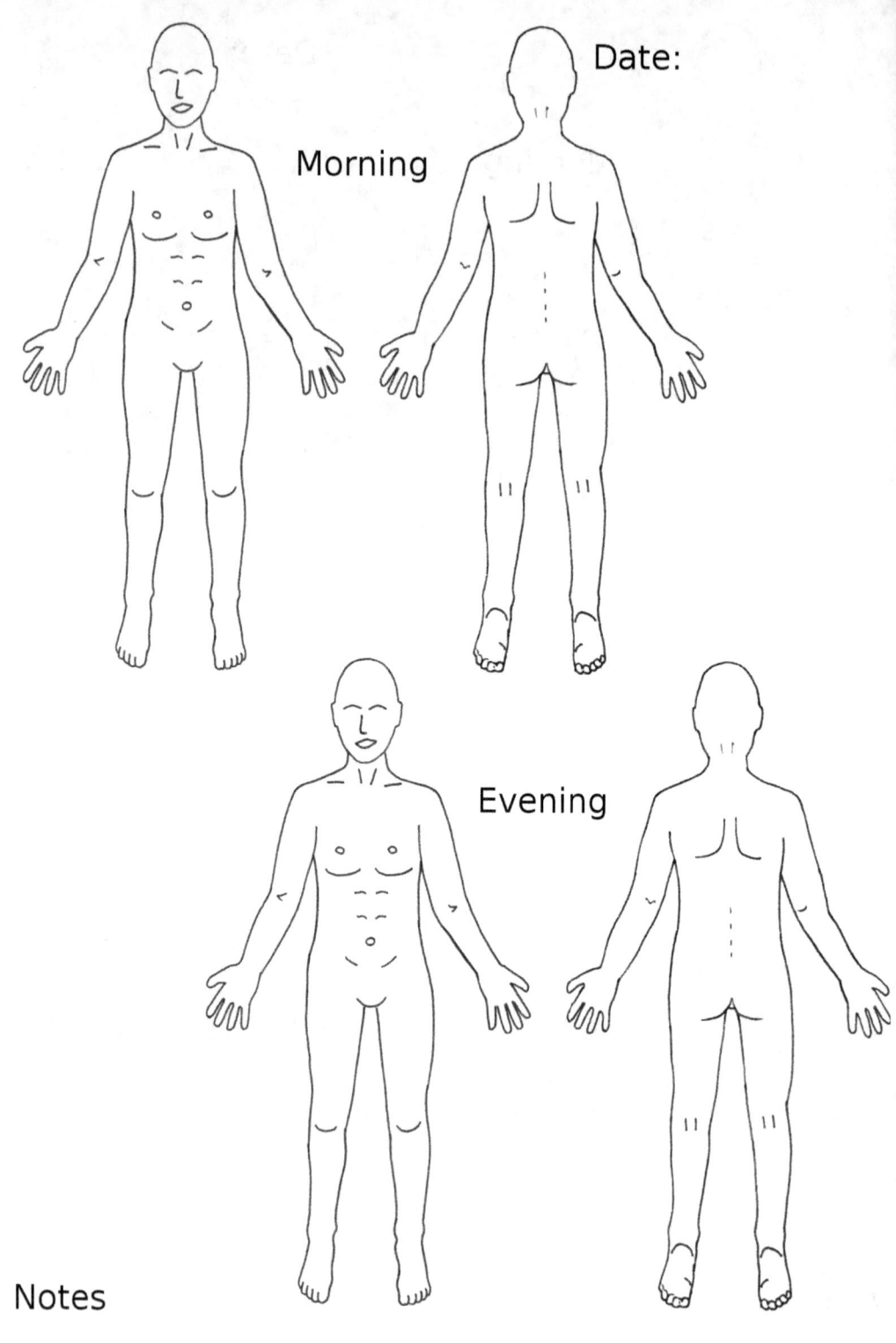

Date:

Morning

Evening

Notes

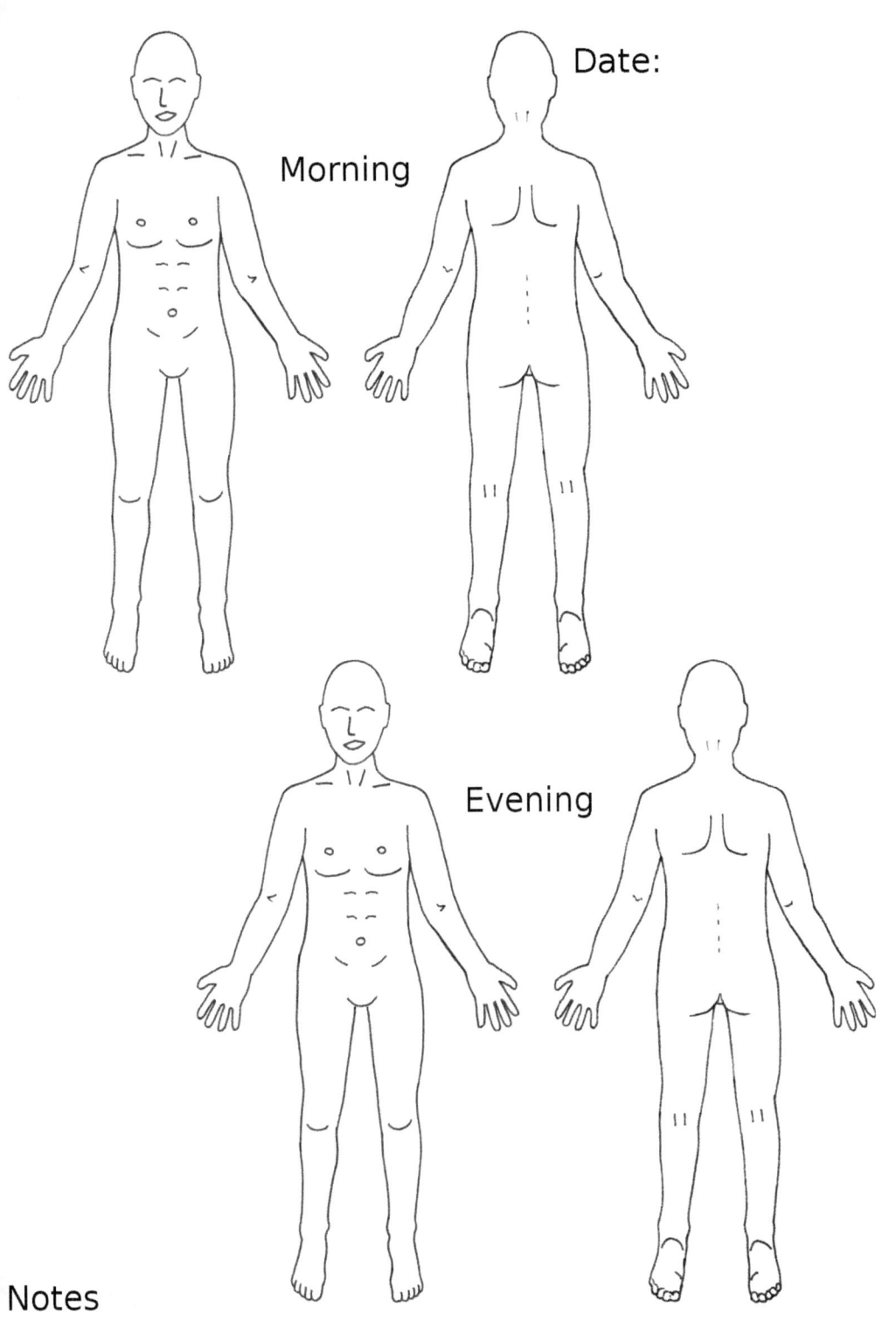

Date:

Morning

Evening

Notes

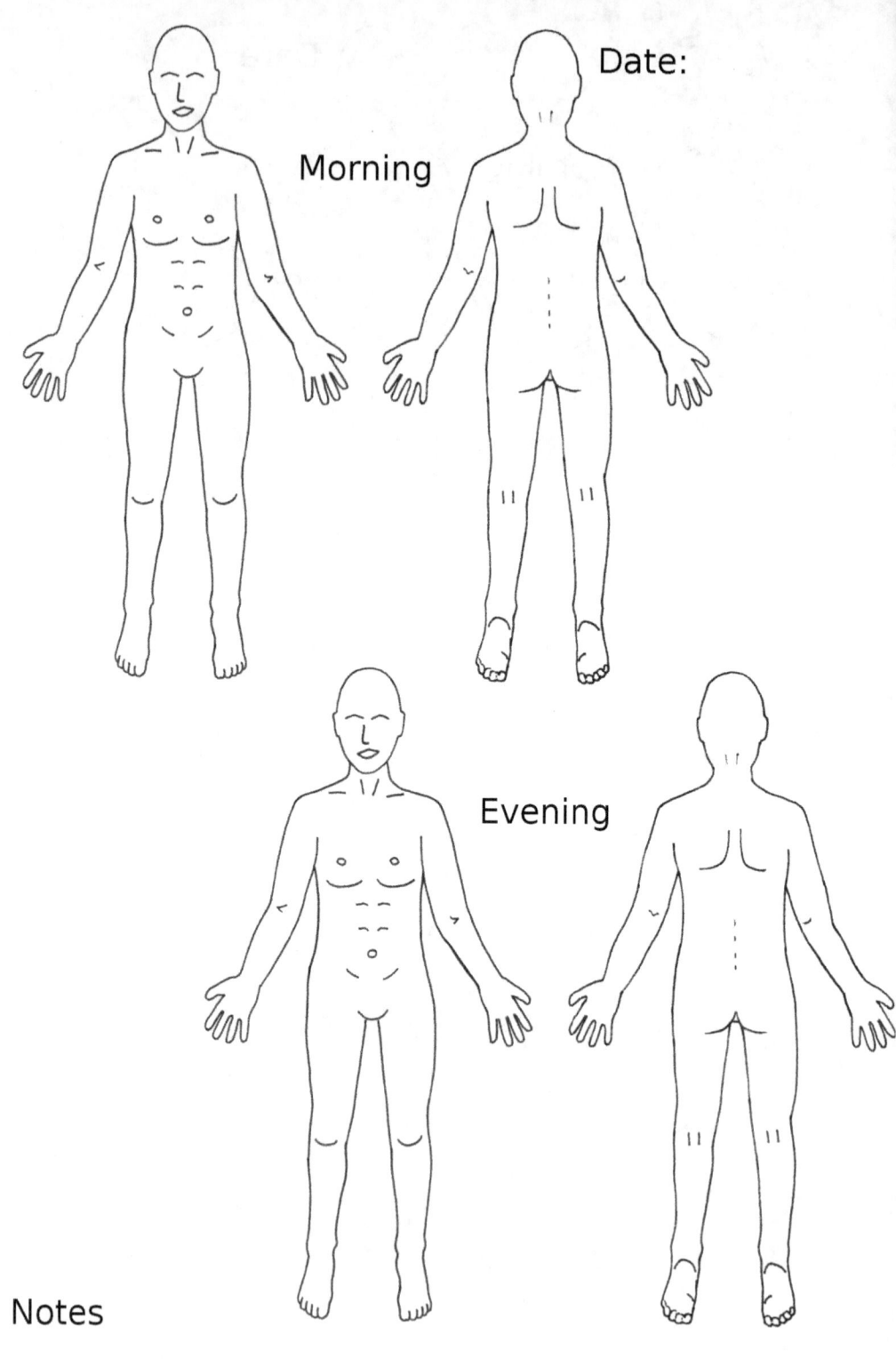

Date:

Morning

Evening

Notes

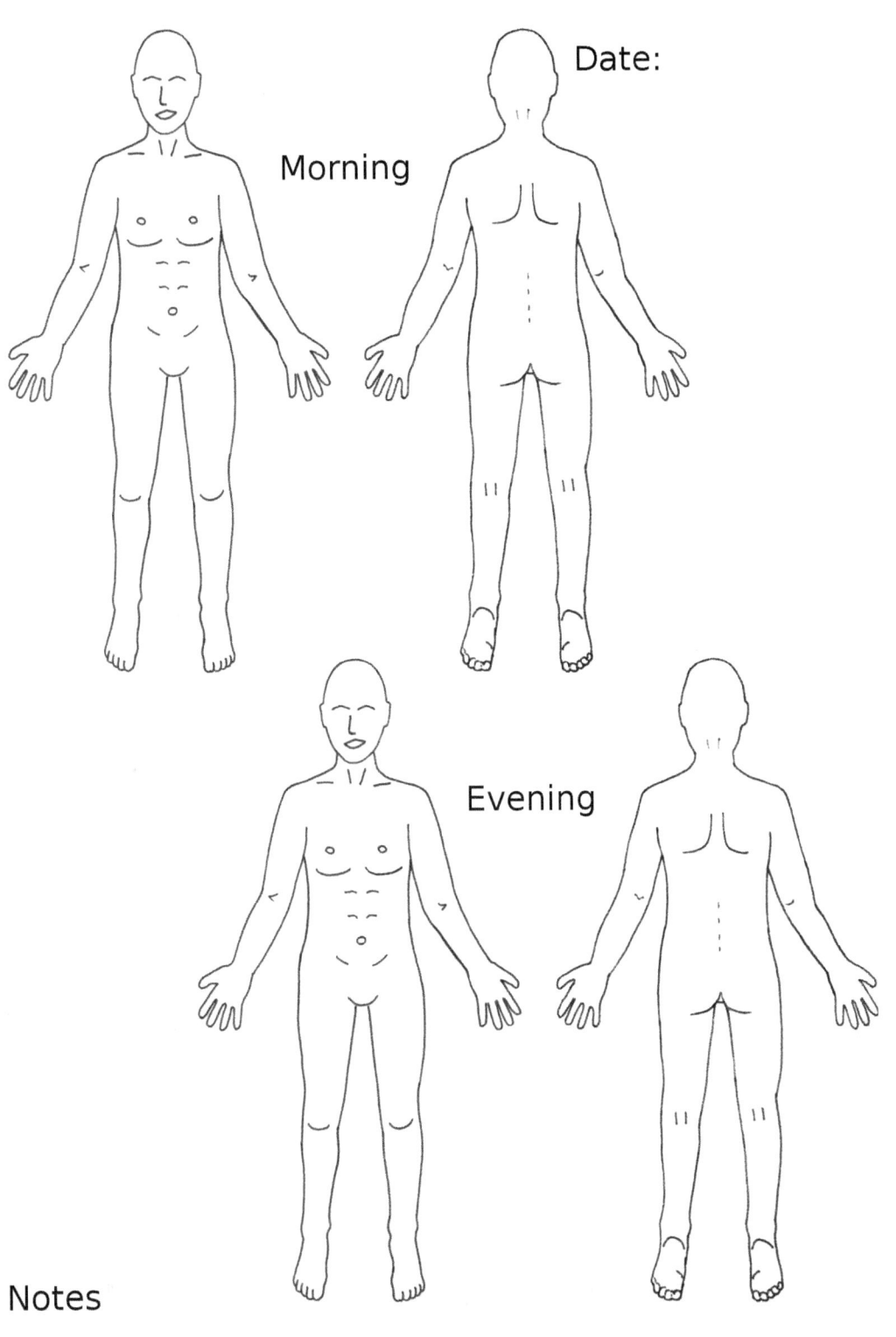

Morning

Date:

Evening

Notes

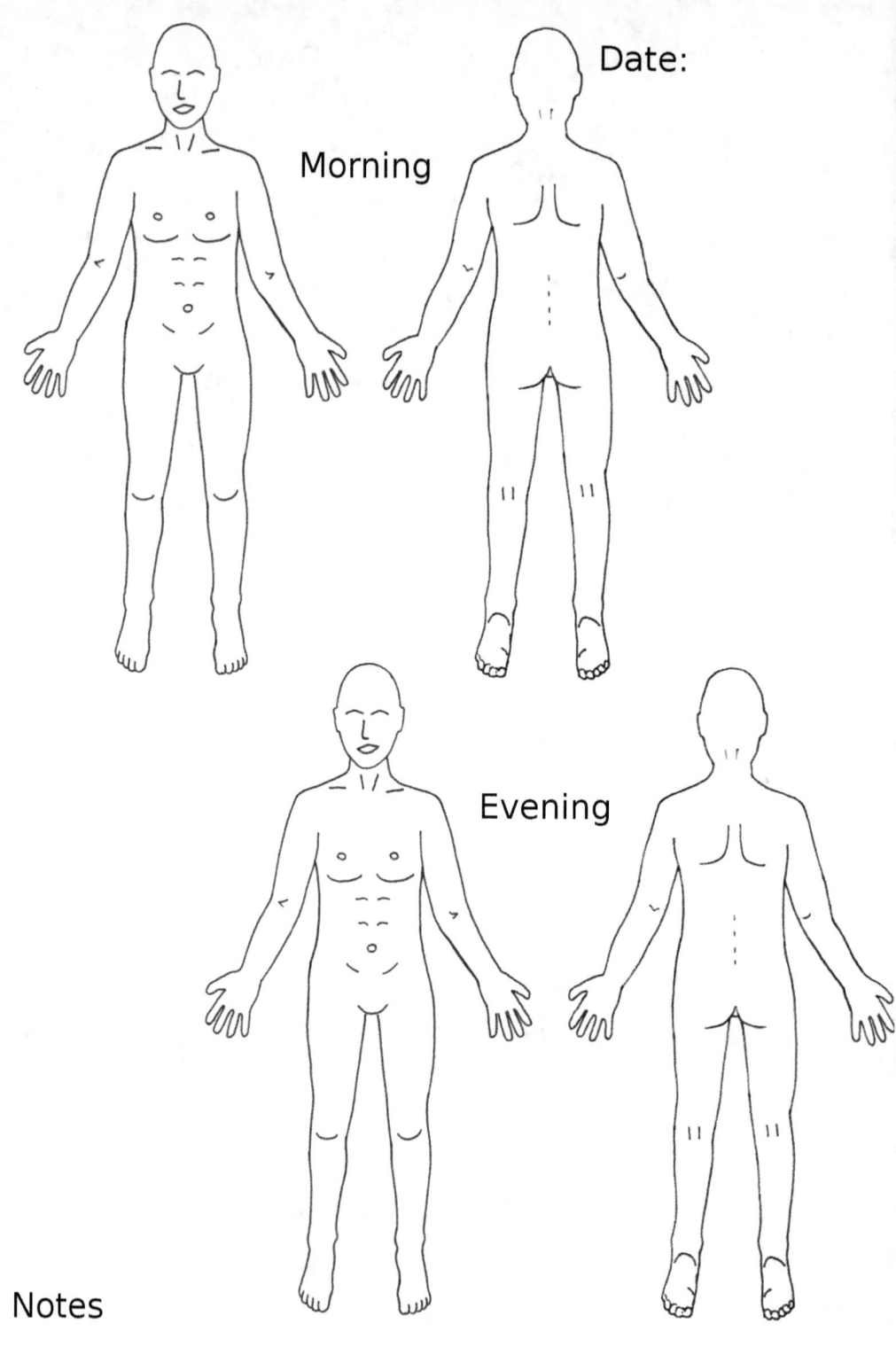

Date:

Morning

Evening

Notes

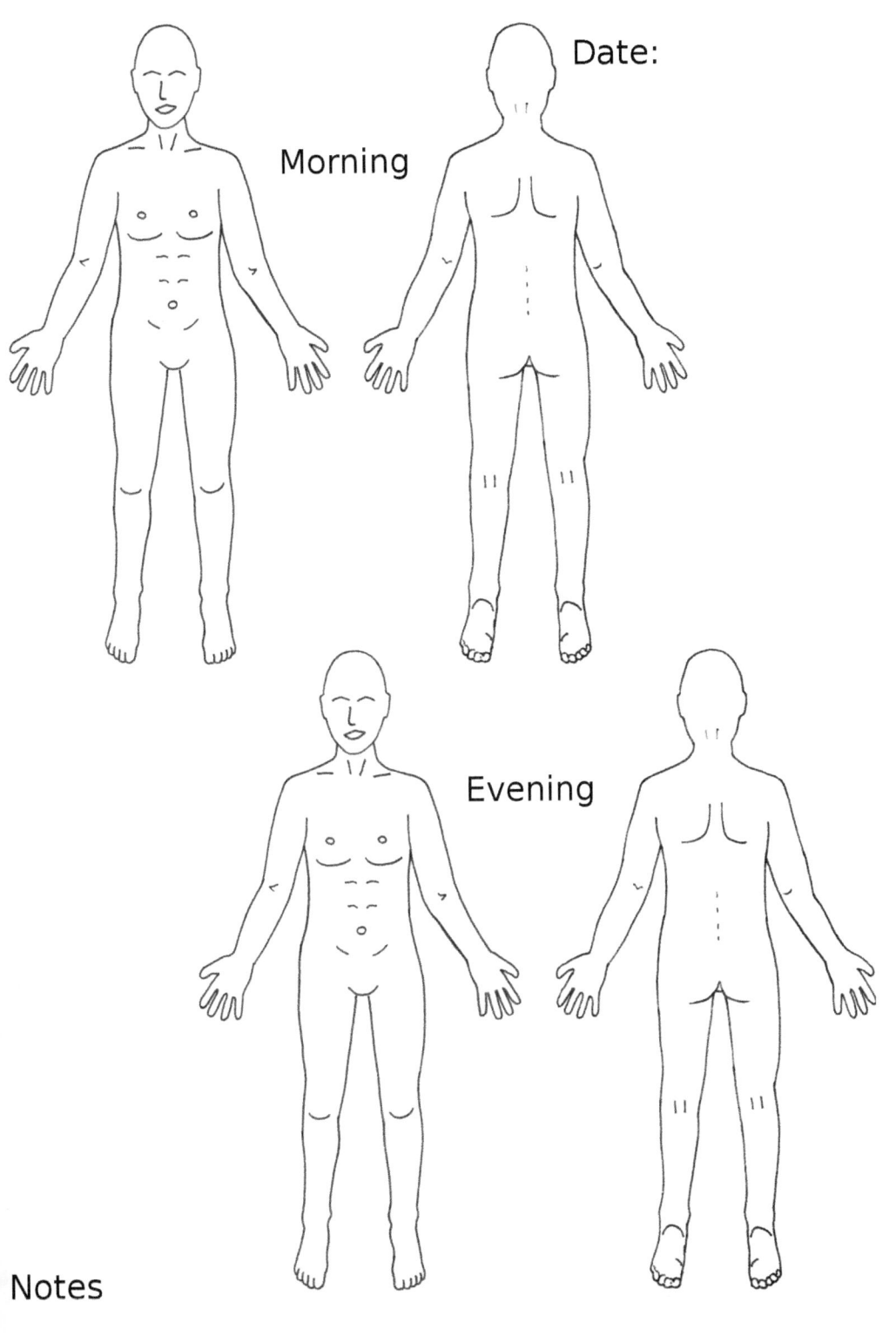

Date:

Morning

Evening

Notes

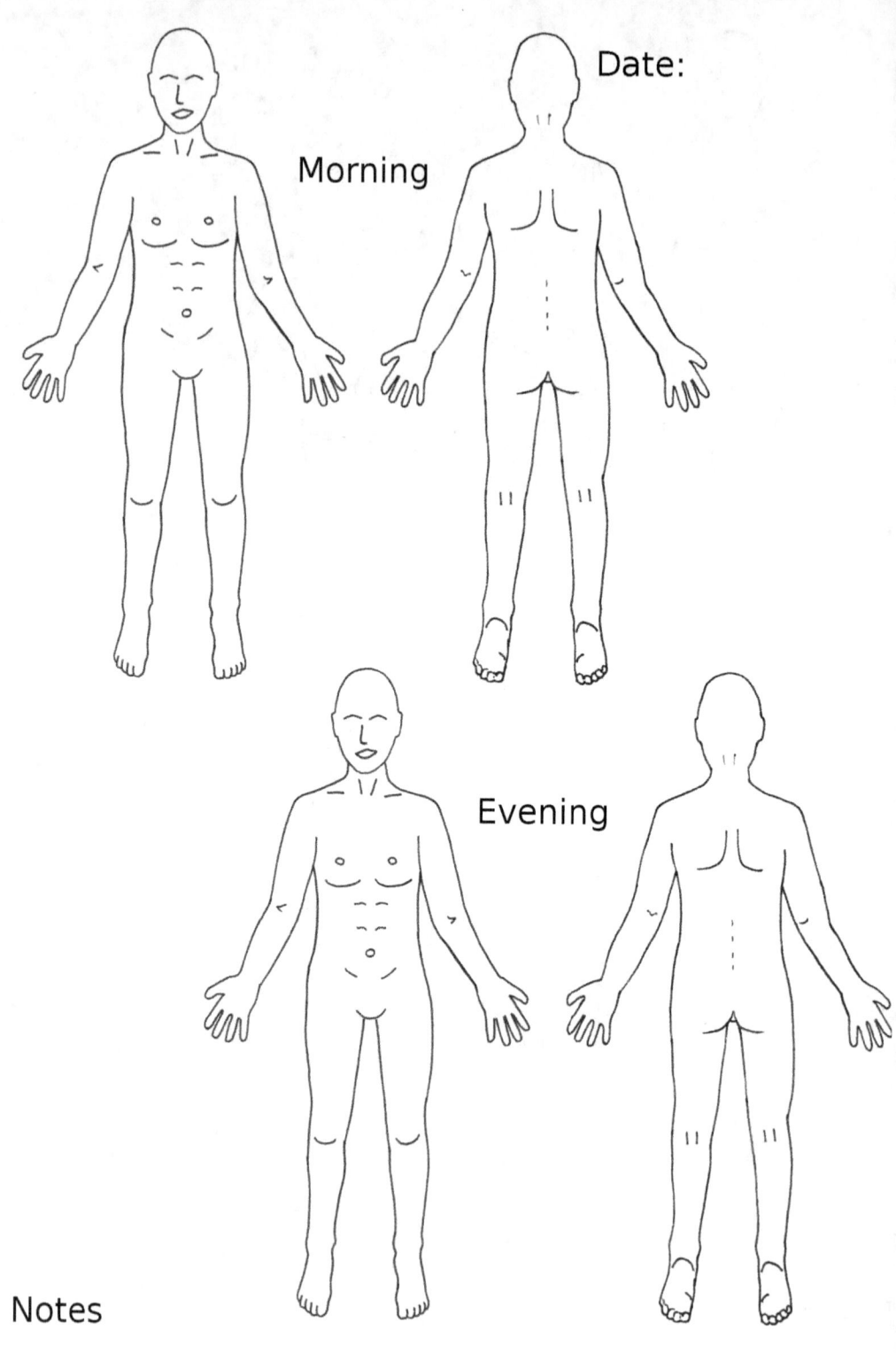

Morning

Date:

Evening

Notes

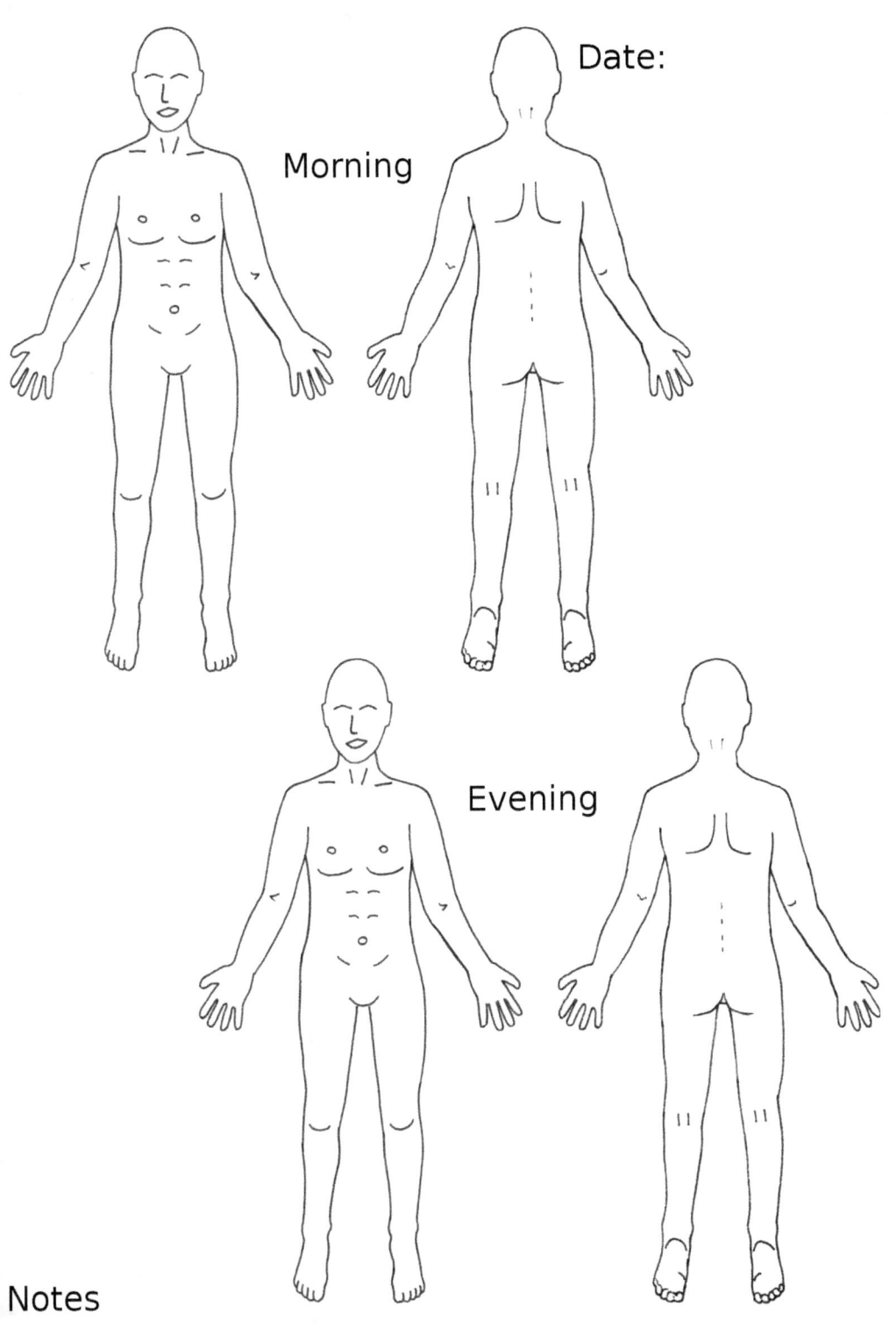

Date:

Morning

Evening

Notes

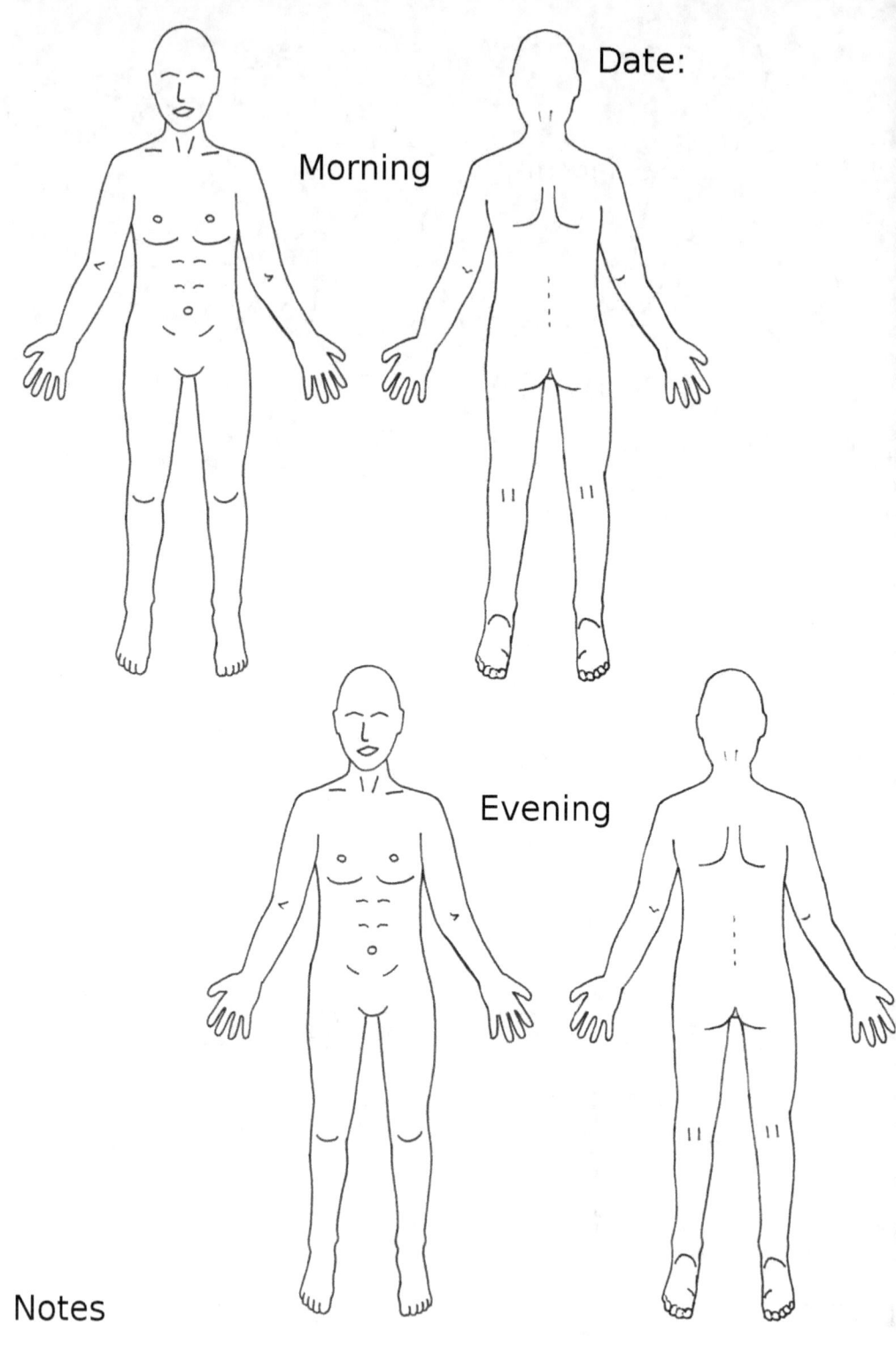

Date:

Morning

Evening

Notes

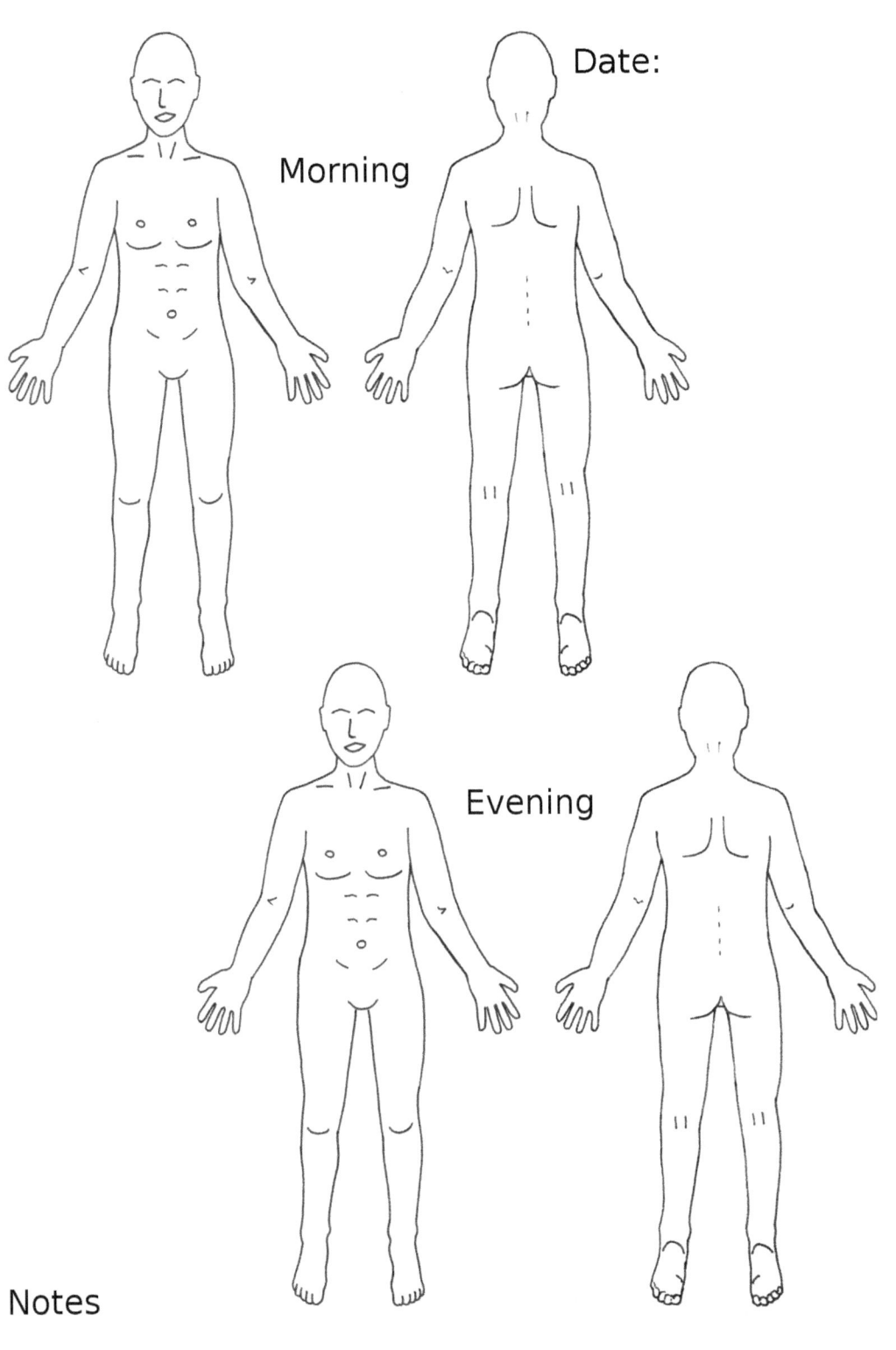

Date:

Morning

Evening

Notes

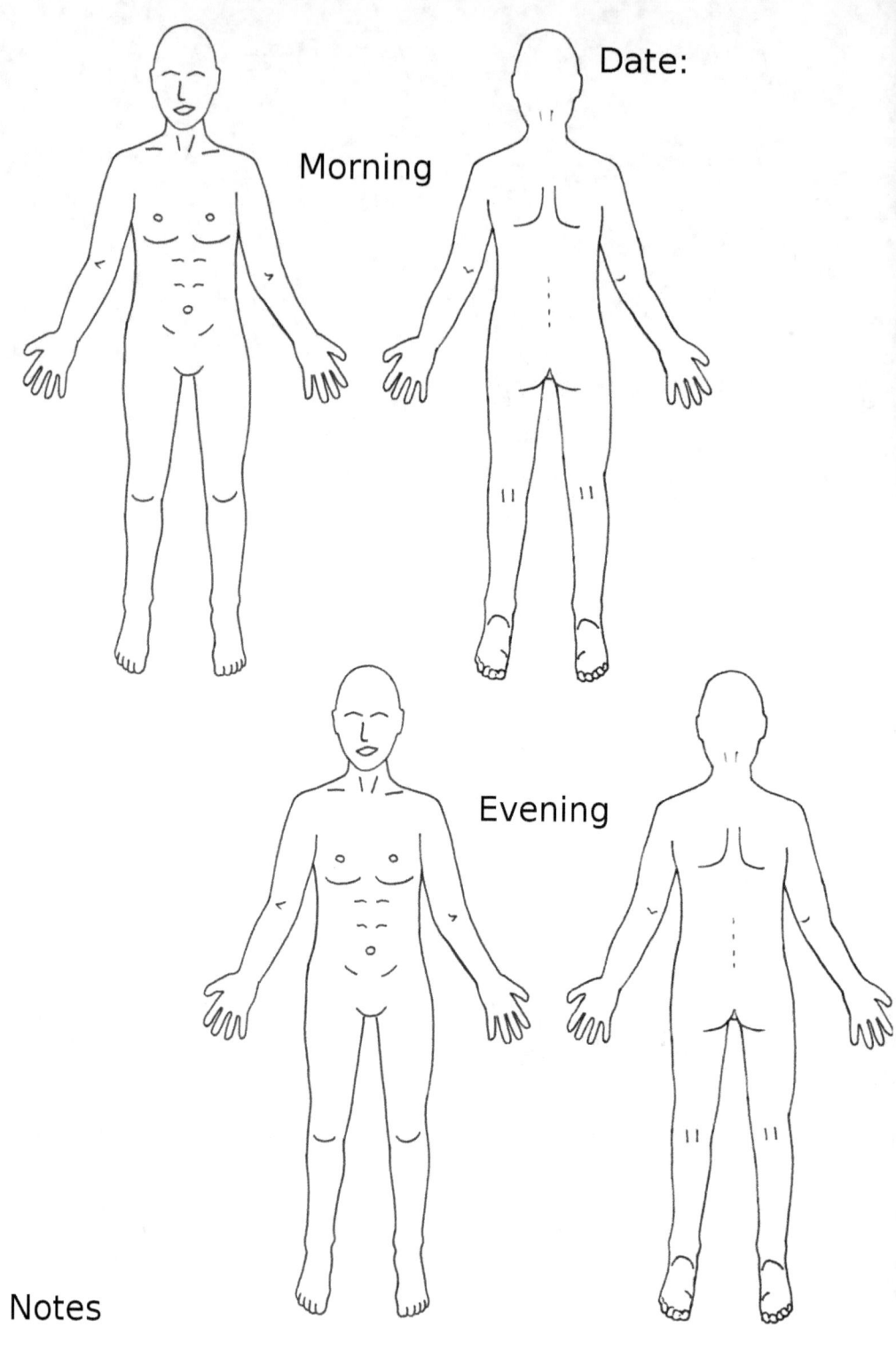

Morning

Date:

Evening

Notes

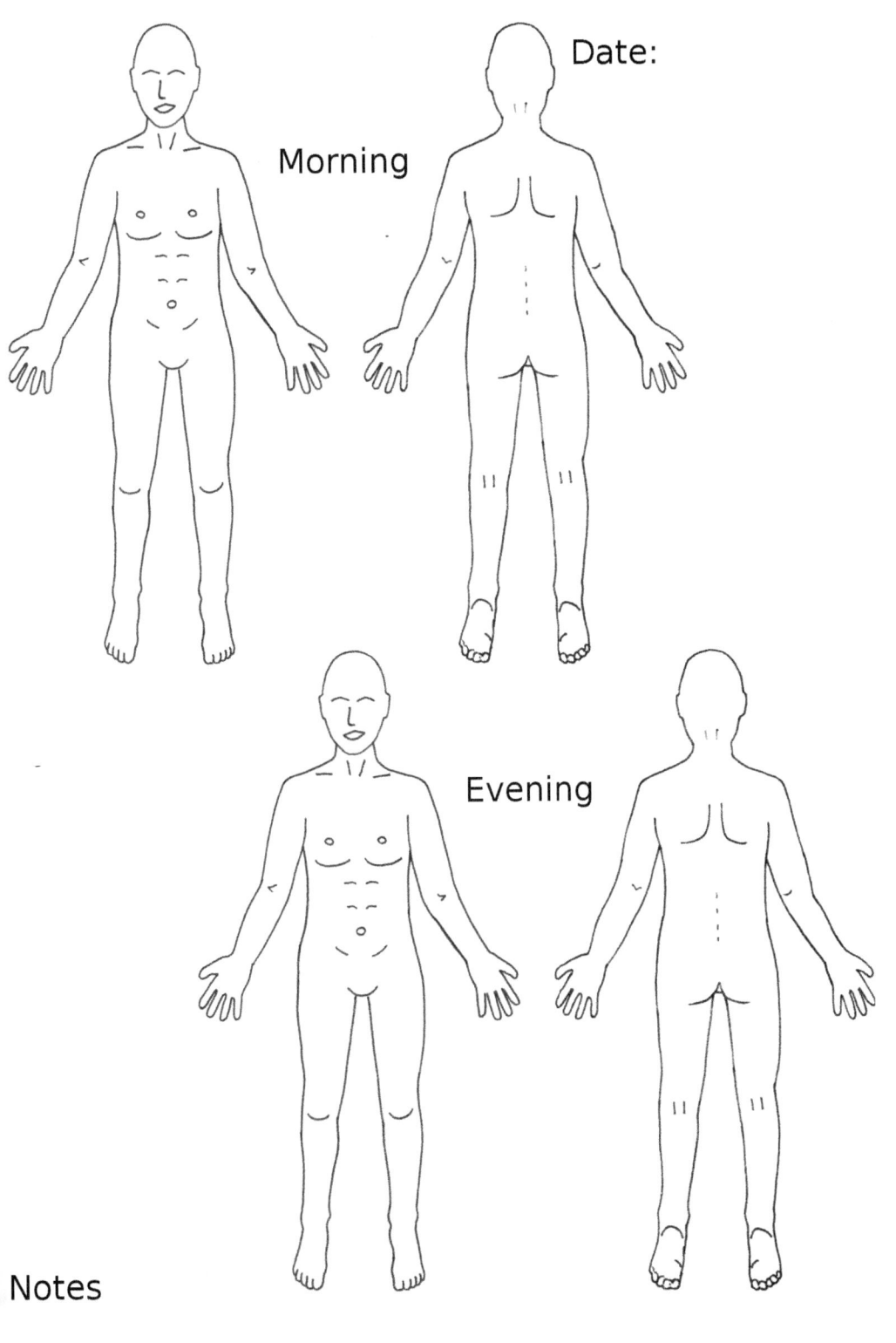

Date:

Morning

Evening

Notes

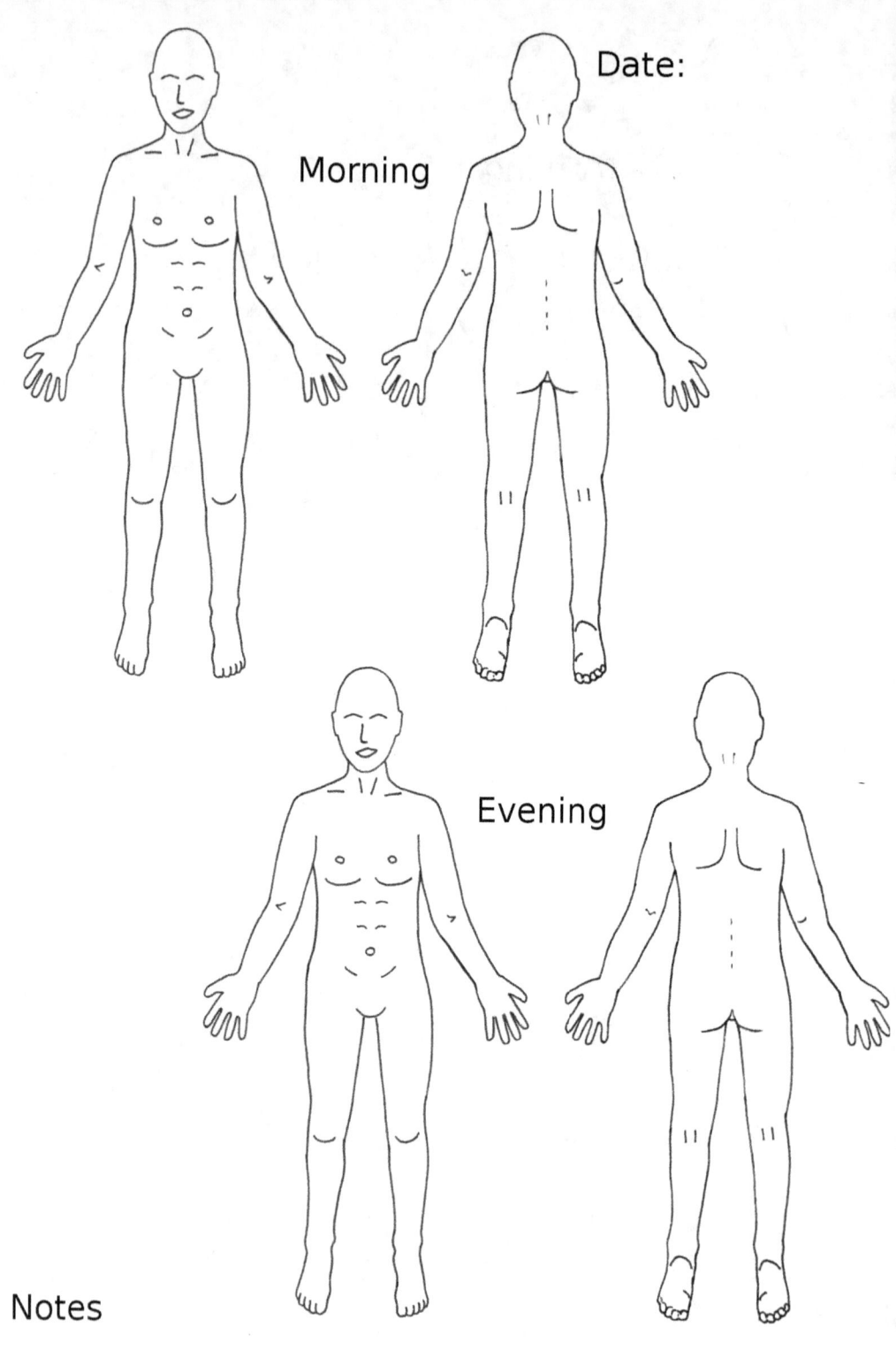

Date:

Morning

Evening

Notes

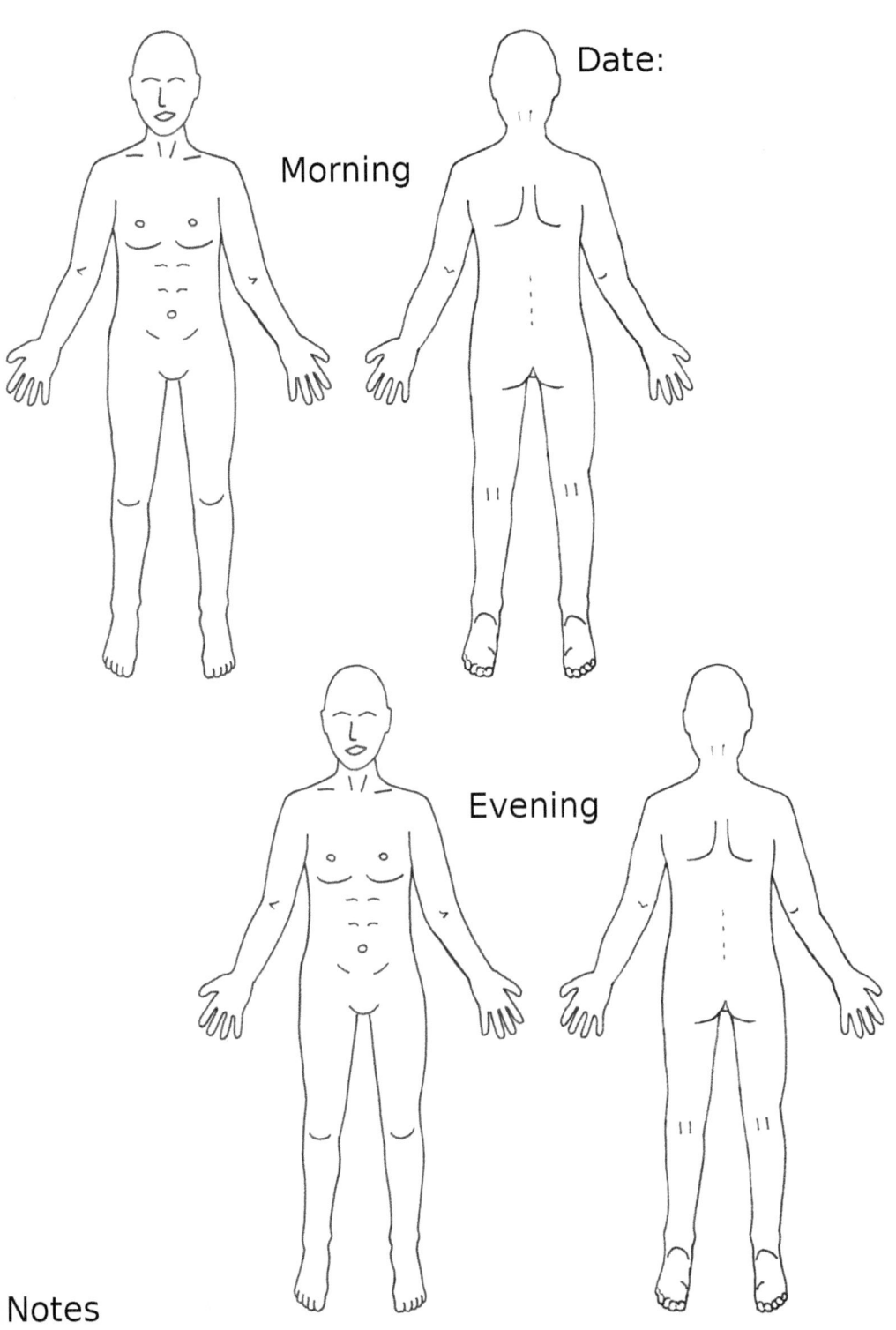

Morning

Date:

Evening

Notes

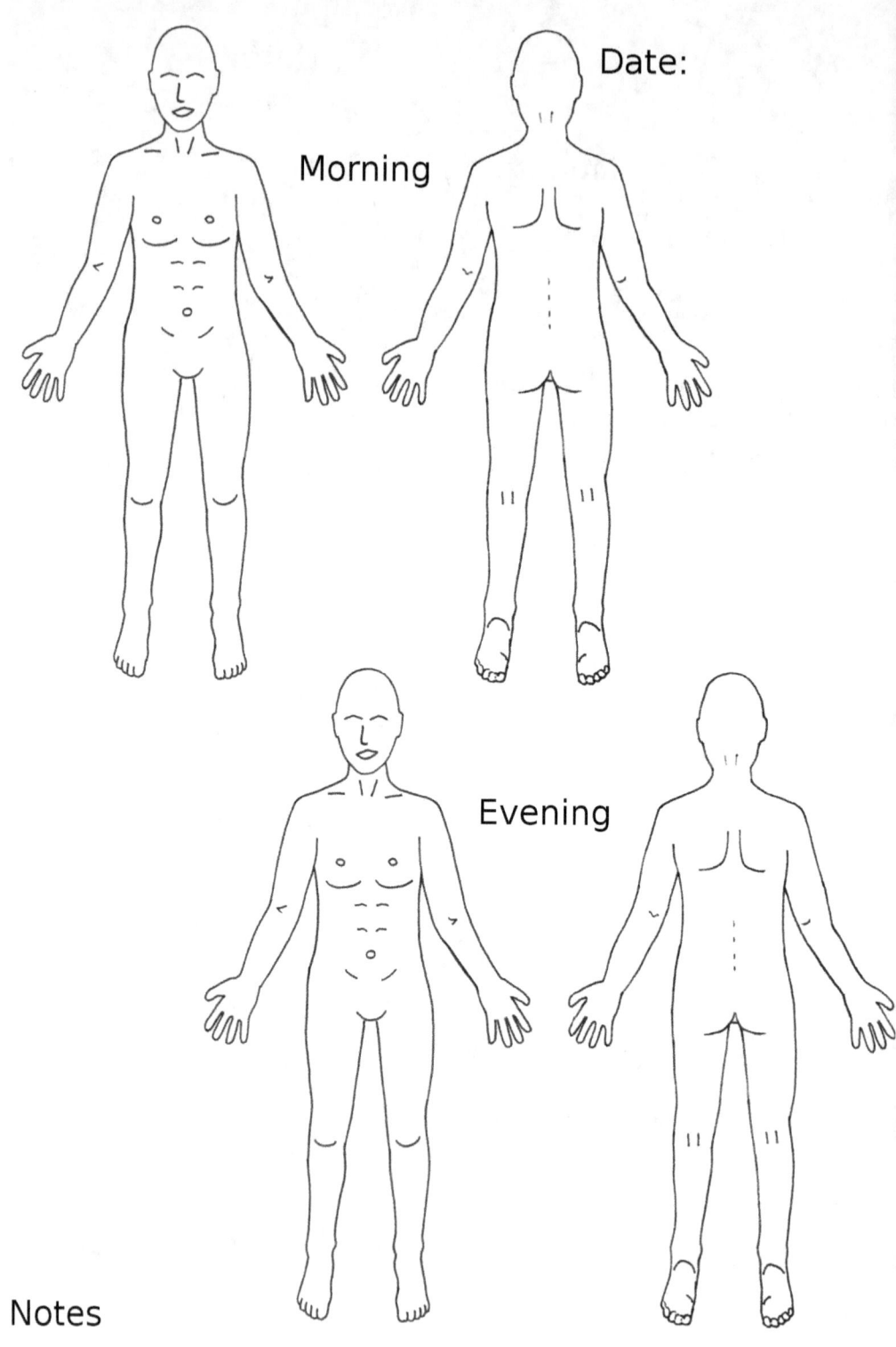

Morning

Date:

Evening

Notes

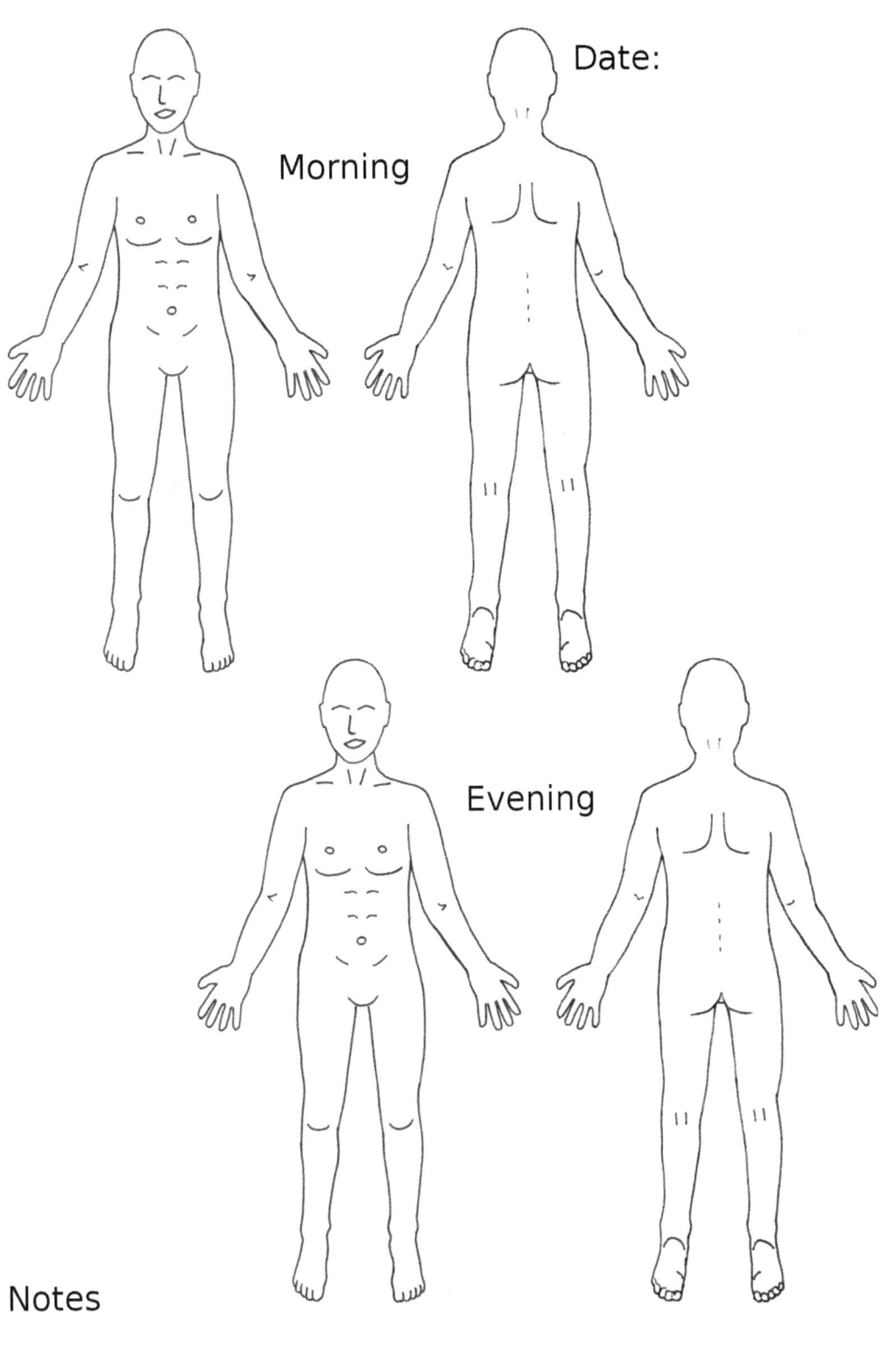

Date:

Morning

Evening

Notes

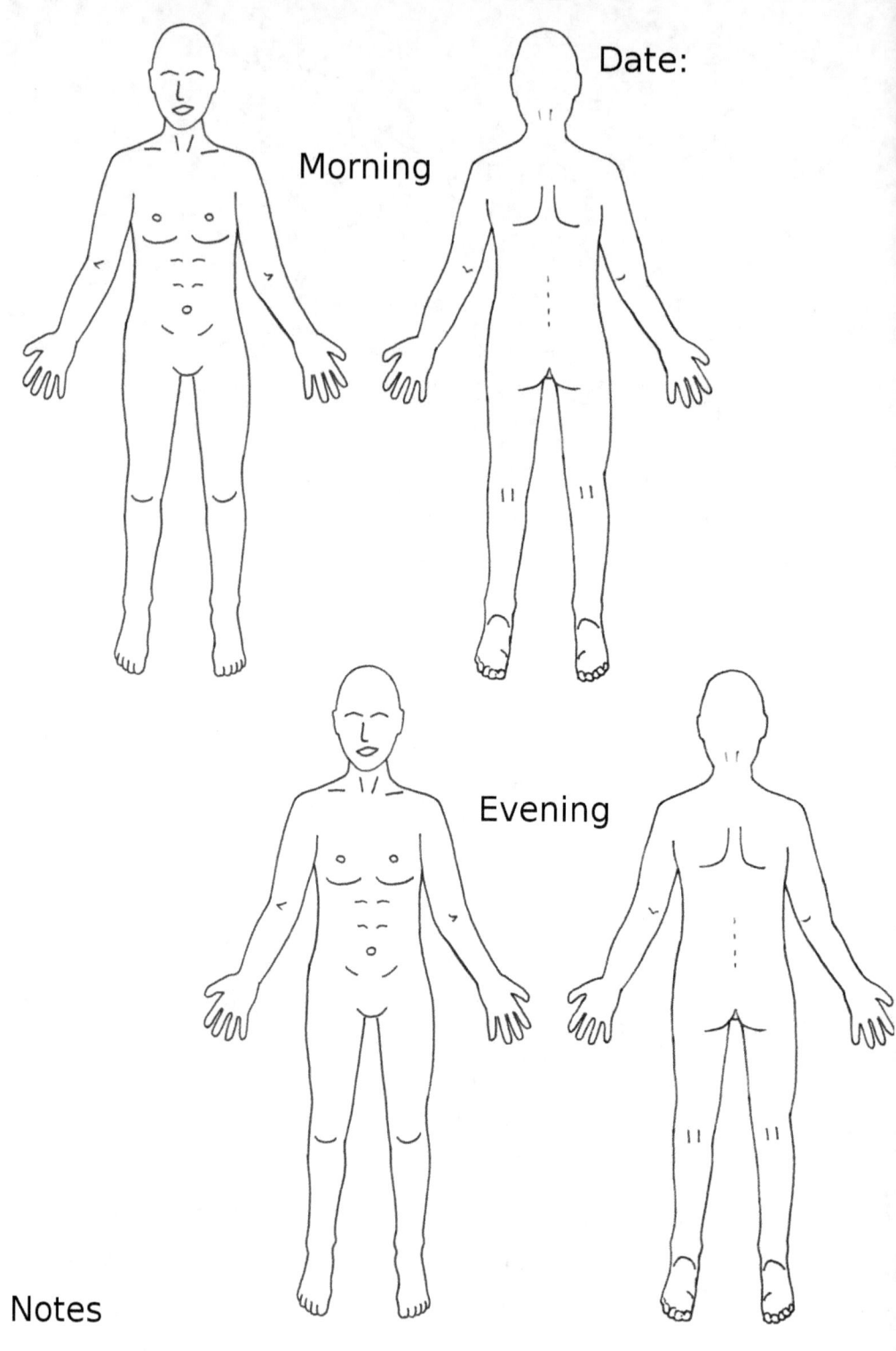

Date:

Morning

Evening

Notes

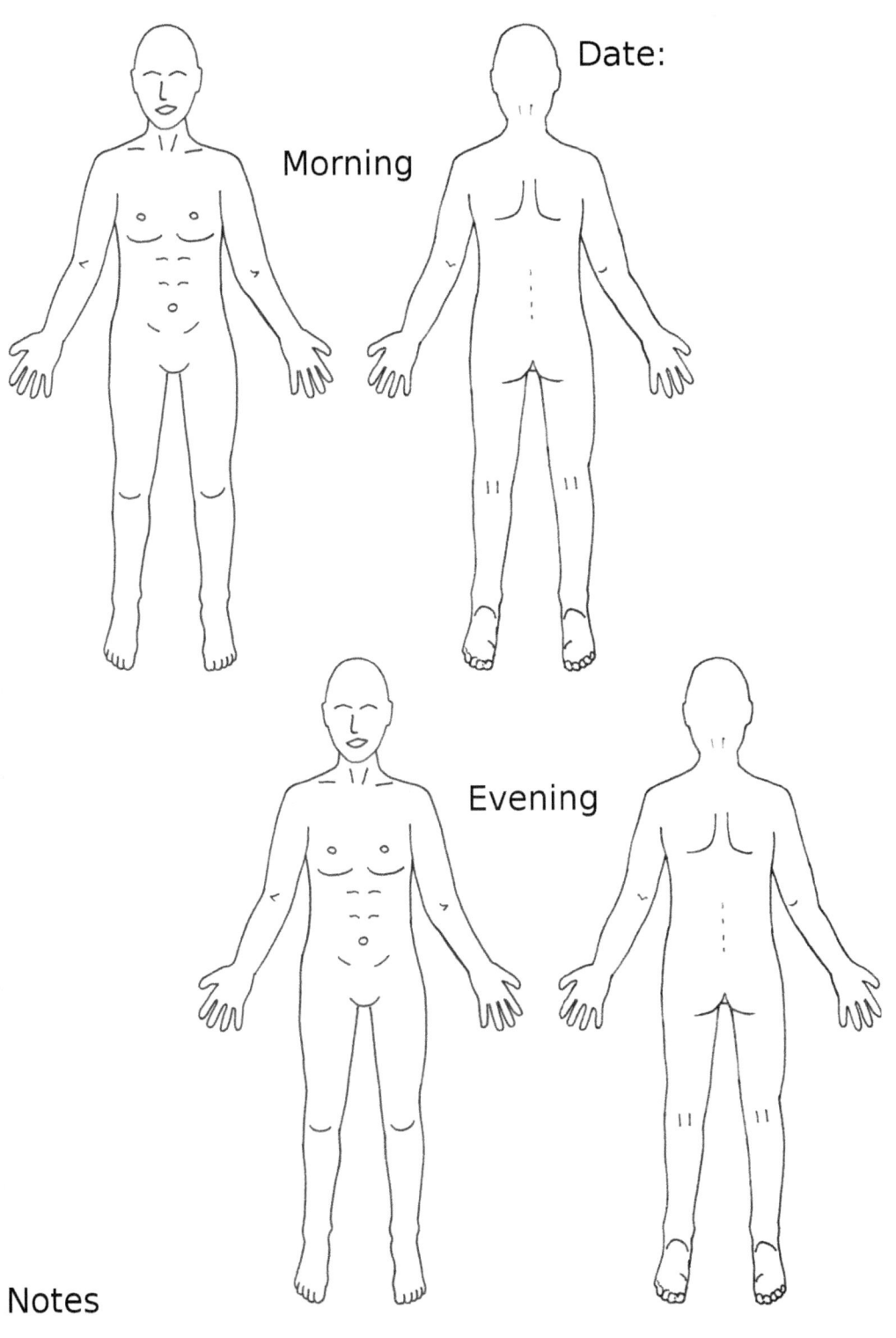

Date:

Morning

Evening

Notes

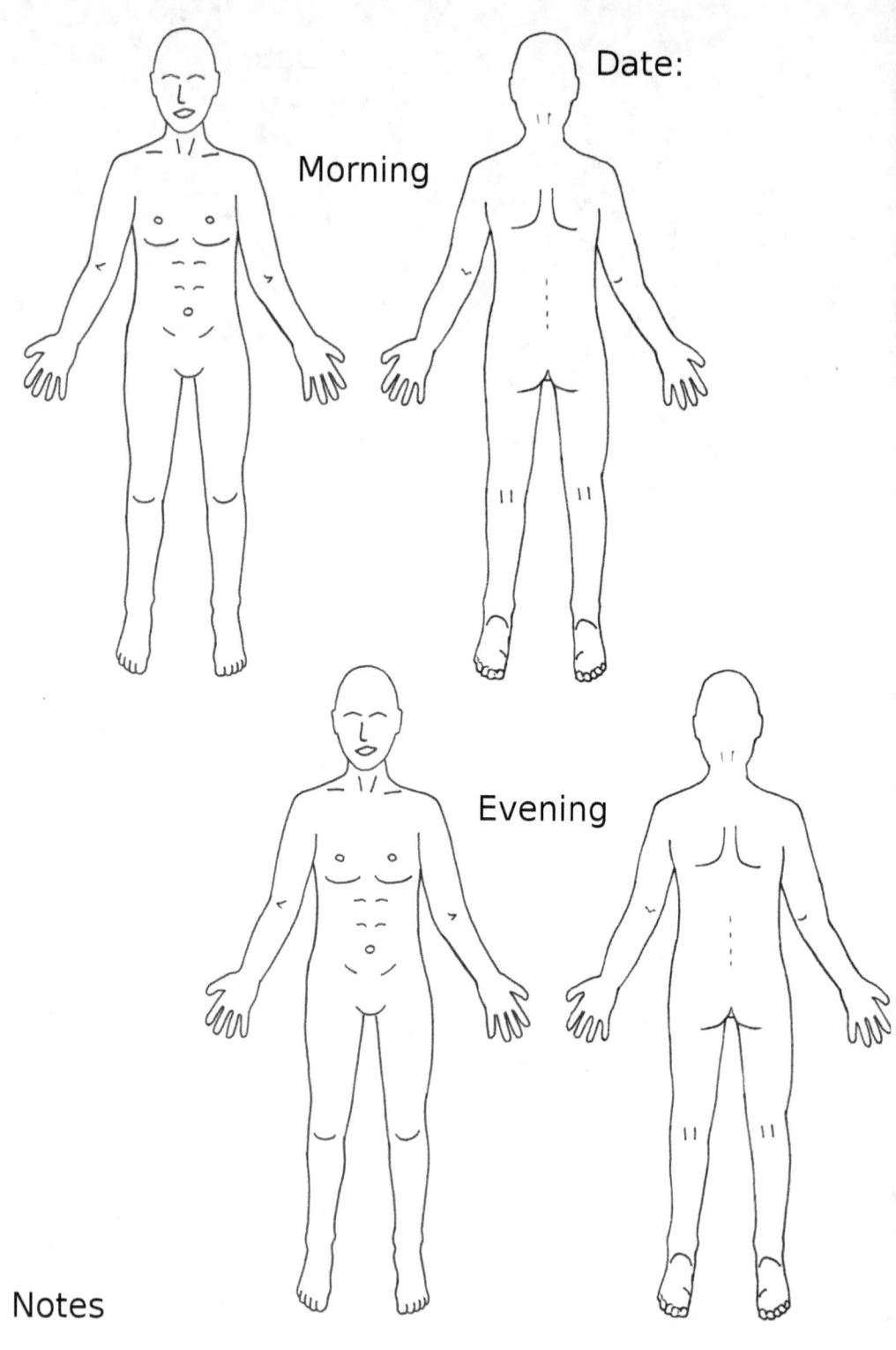

Date:

Morning

Evening

Notes

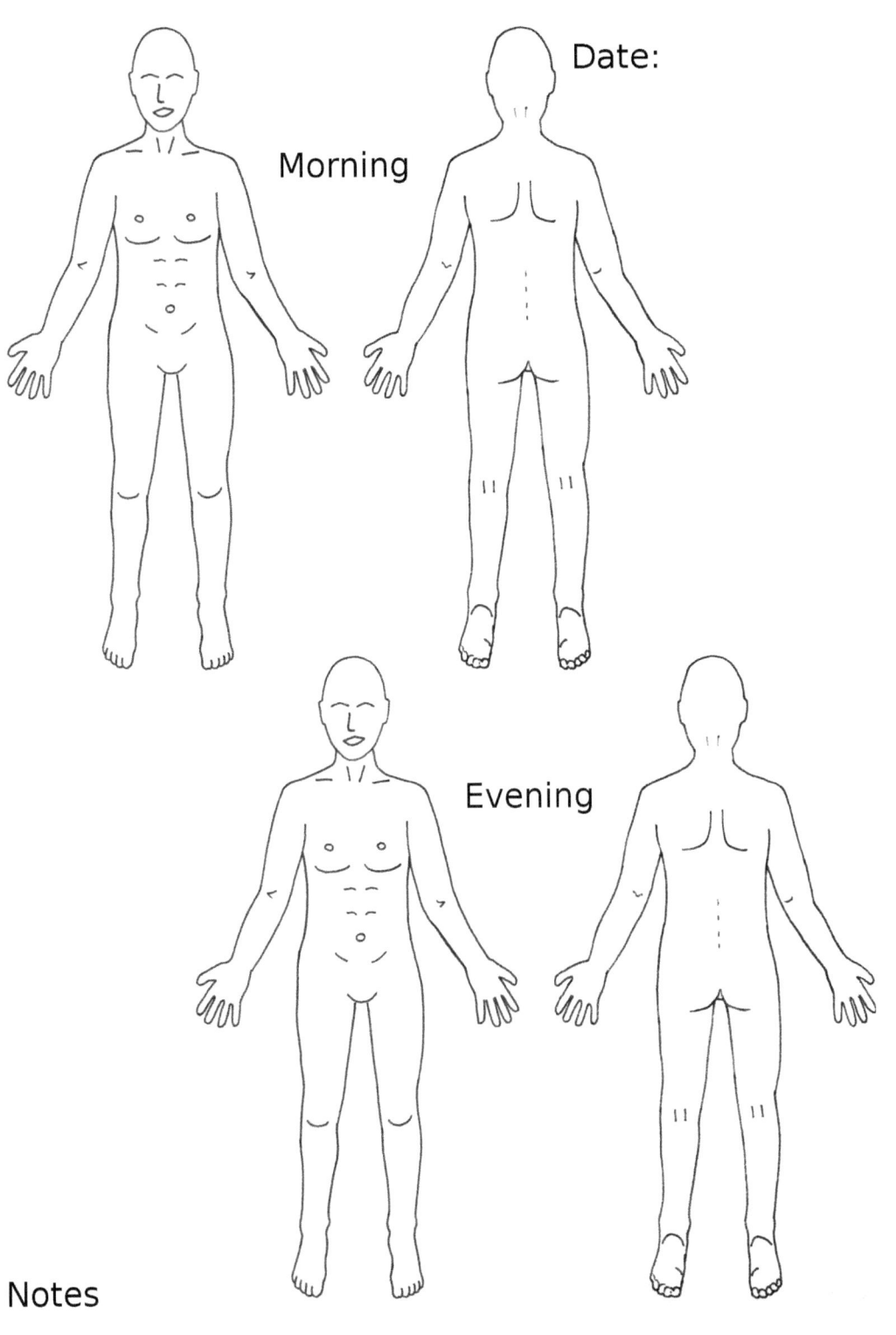

Date:

Morning

Evening

Notes

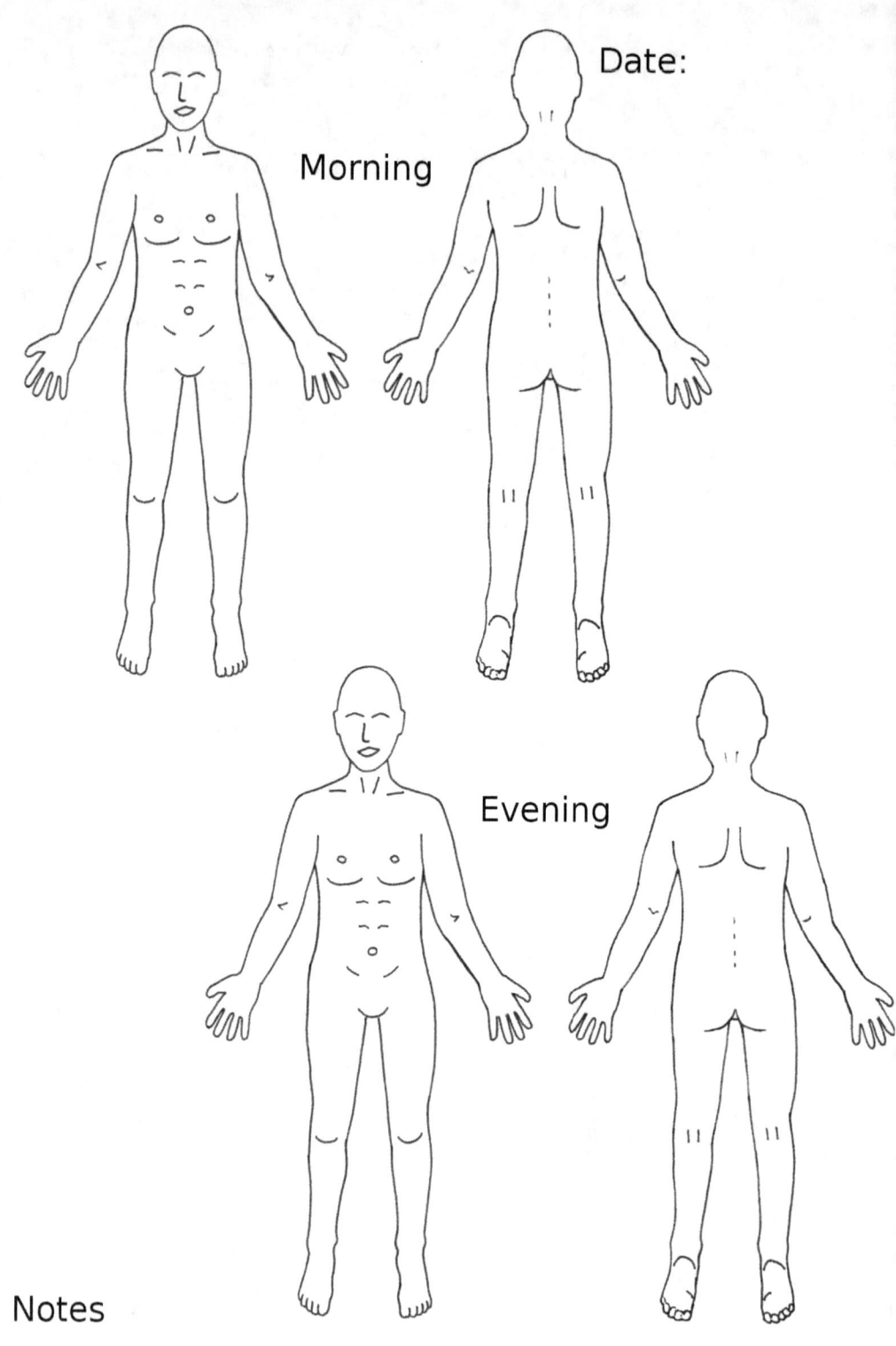

Date:

Morning

Evening

Notes

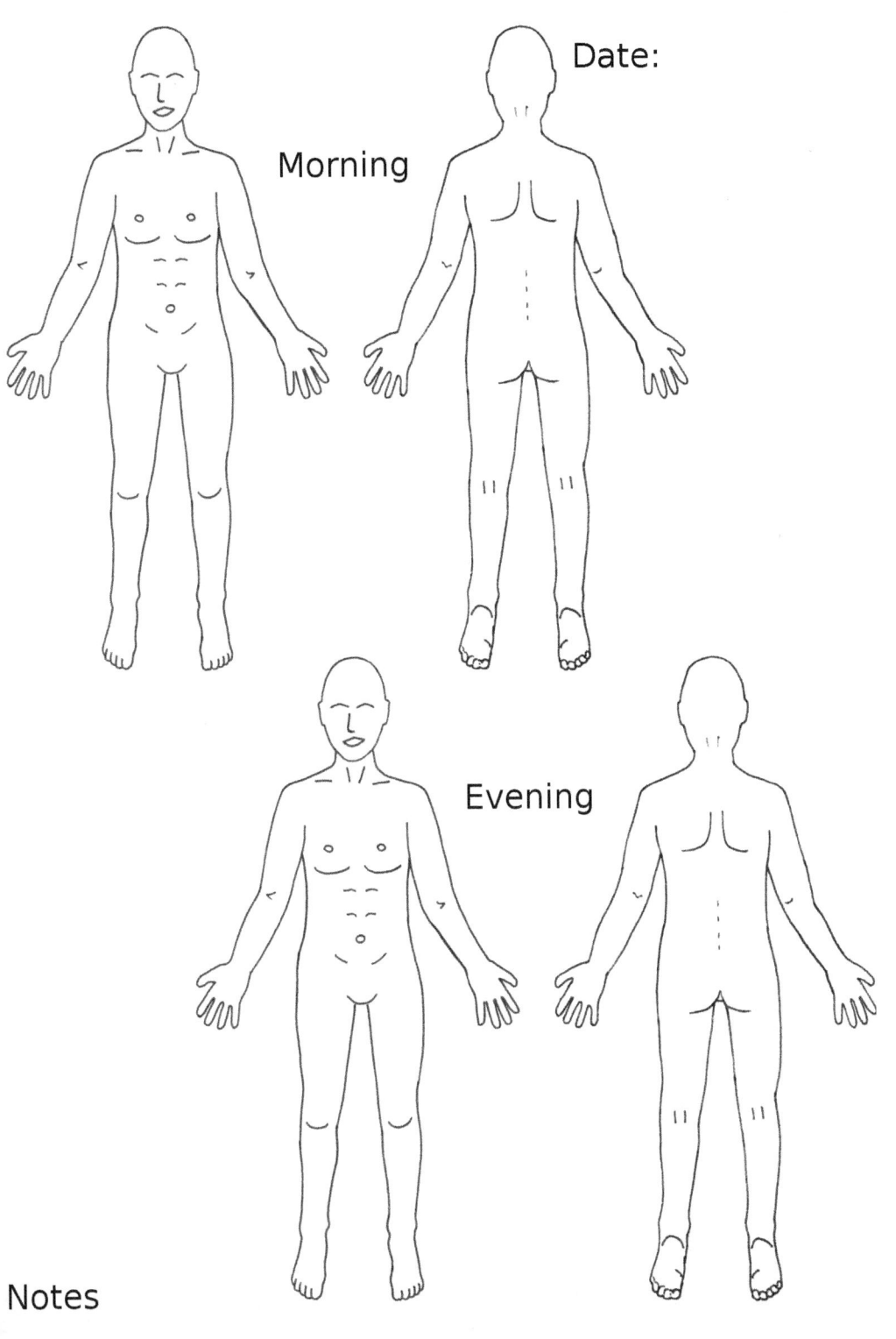

Morning

Date:

Evening

Notes

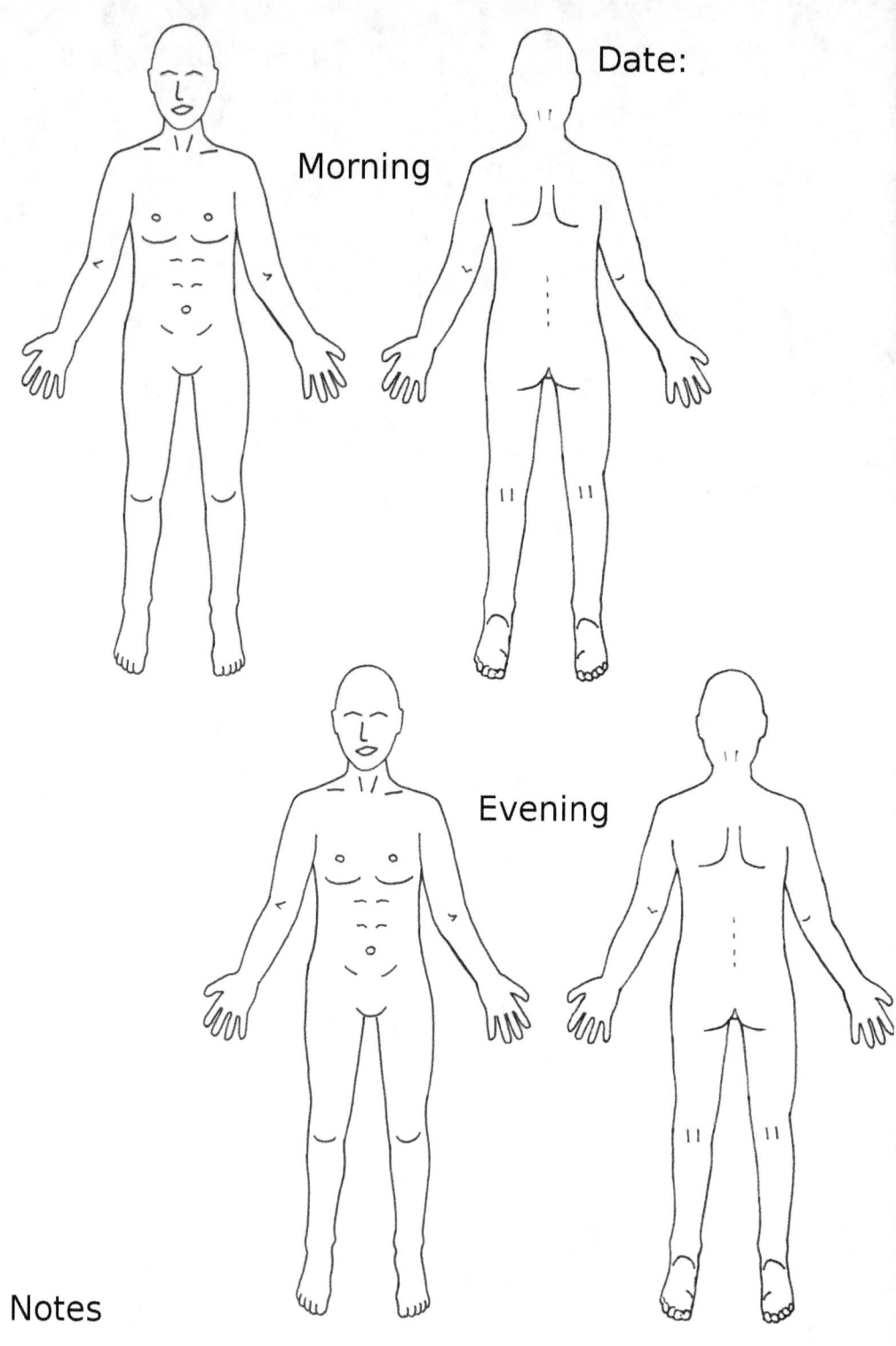

Date:

Morning

Evening

Notes

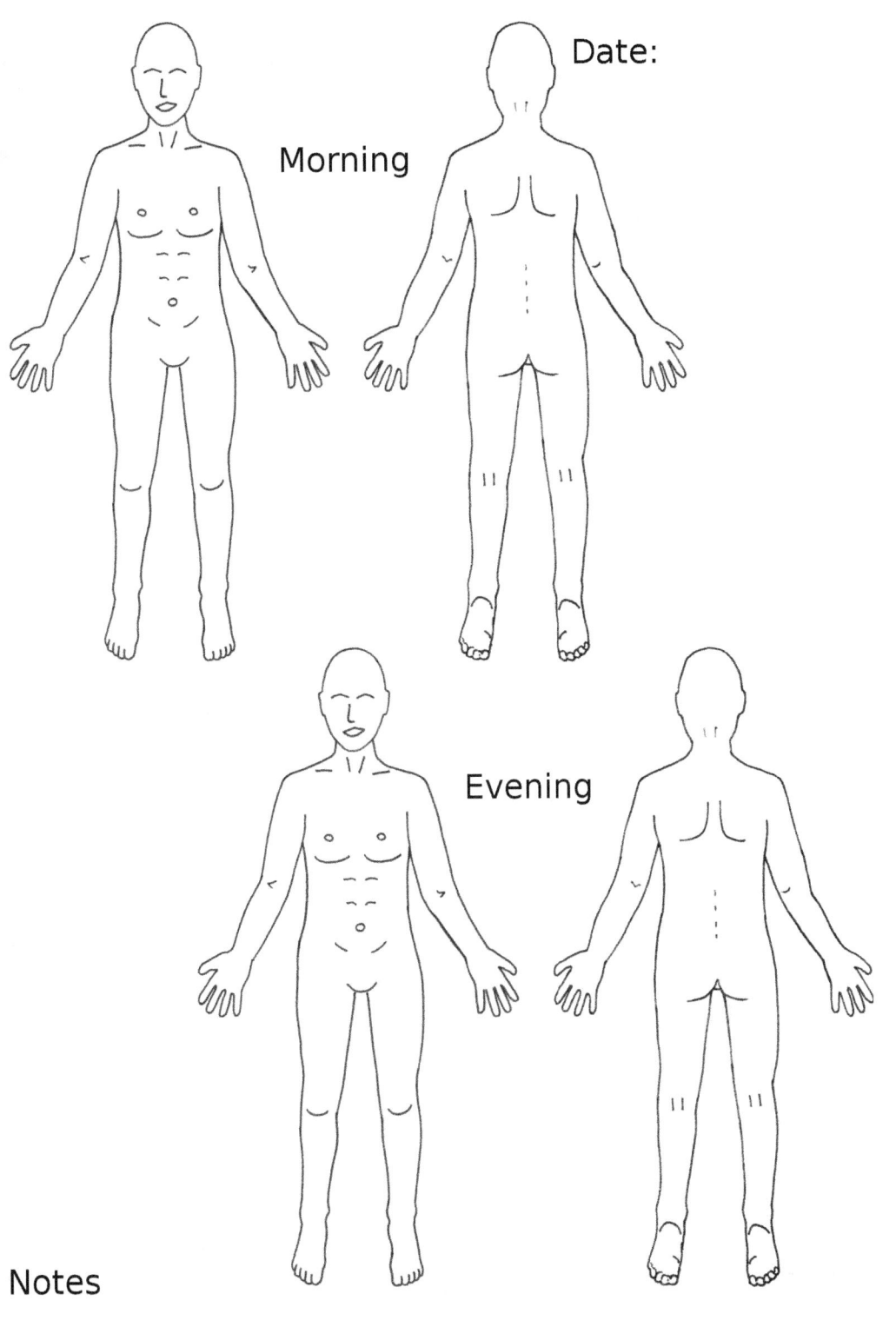

Morning

Date:

Evening

Notes

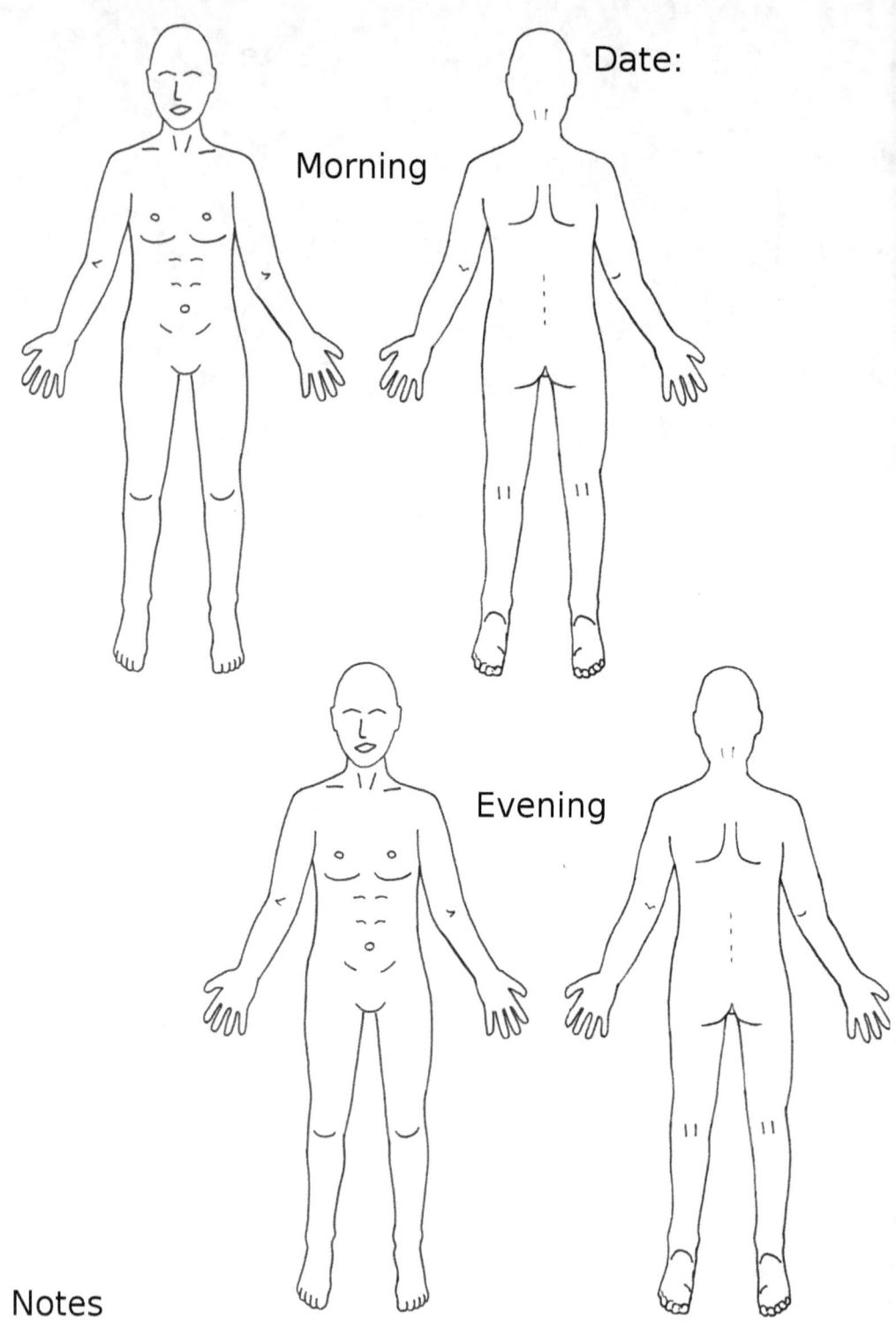

Morning

Date:

Evening

Notes

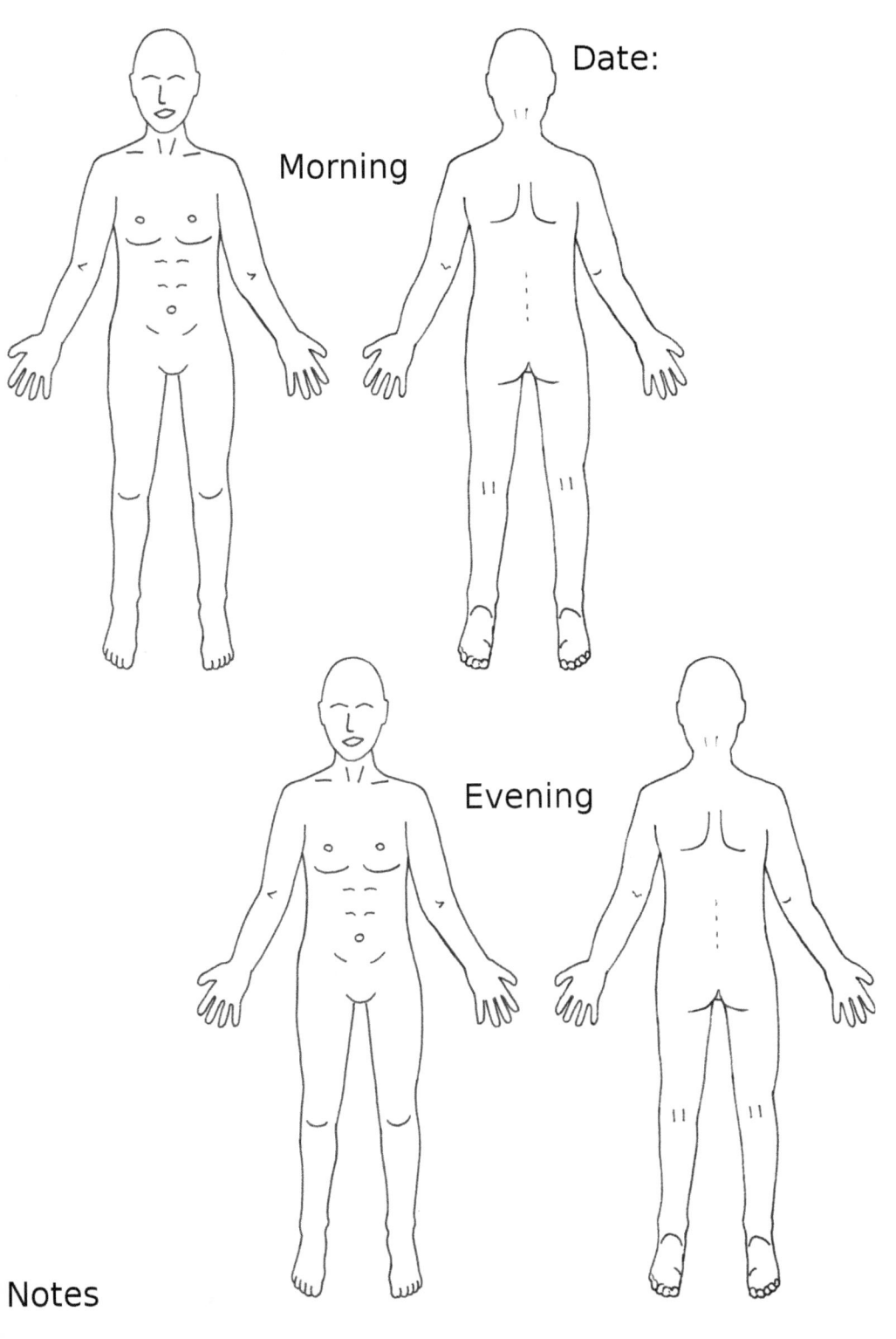

Morning

Date:

Evening

Notes

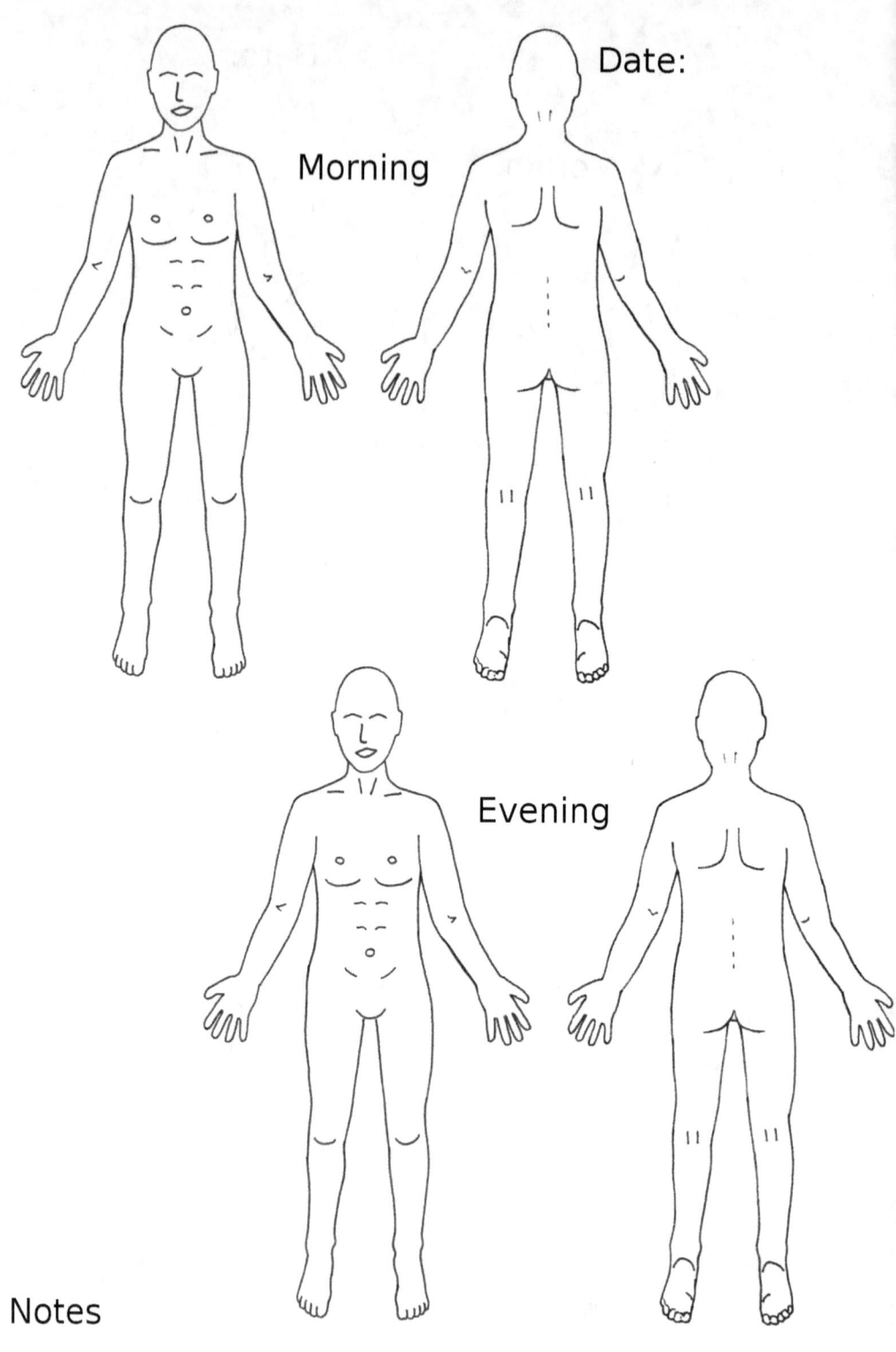

Morning

Date:

Evening

Notes

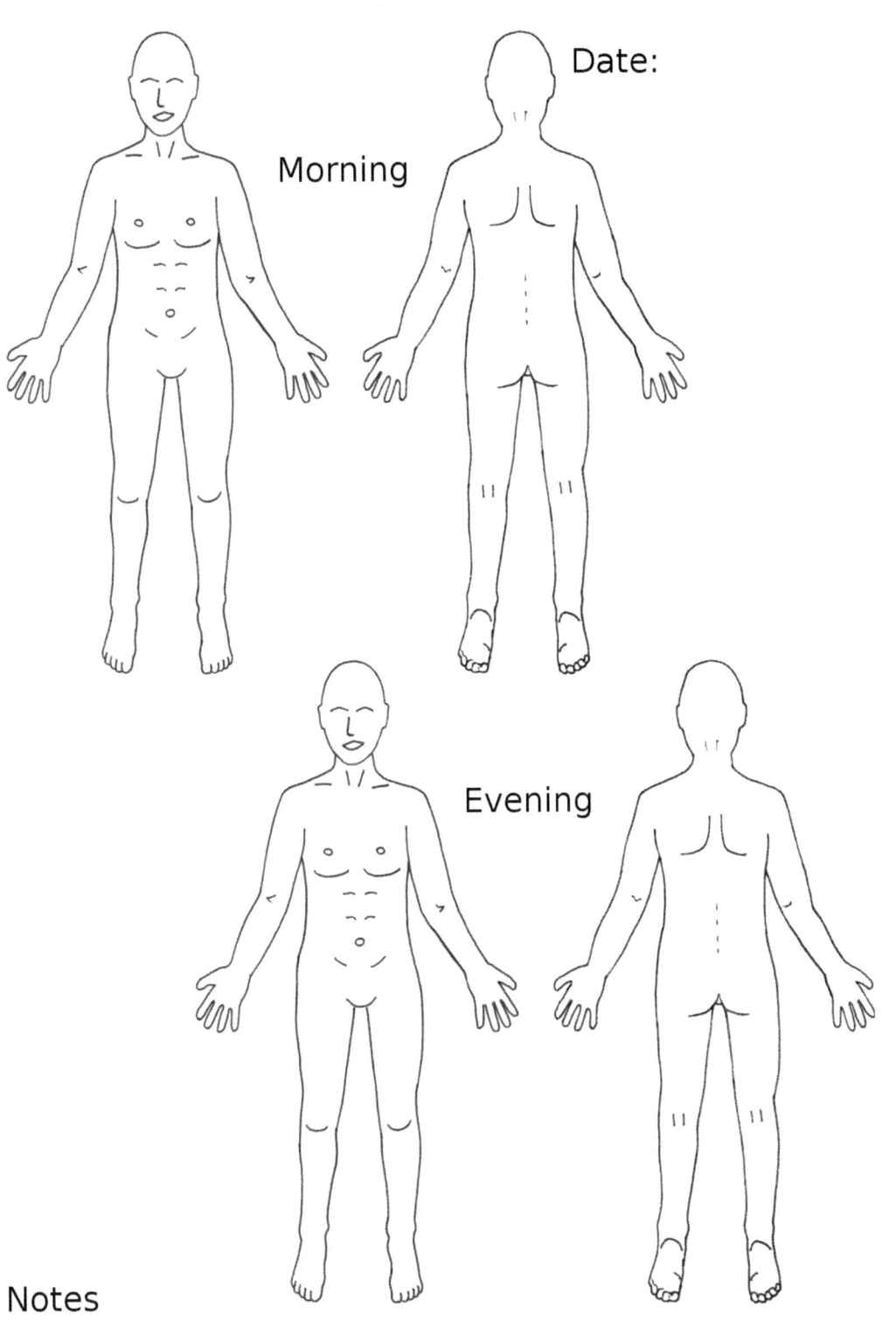

Date:

Morning

Evening

Notes

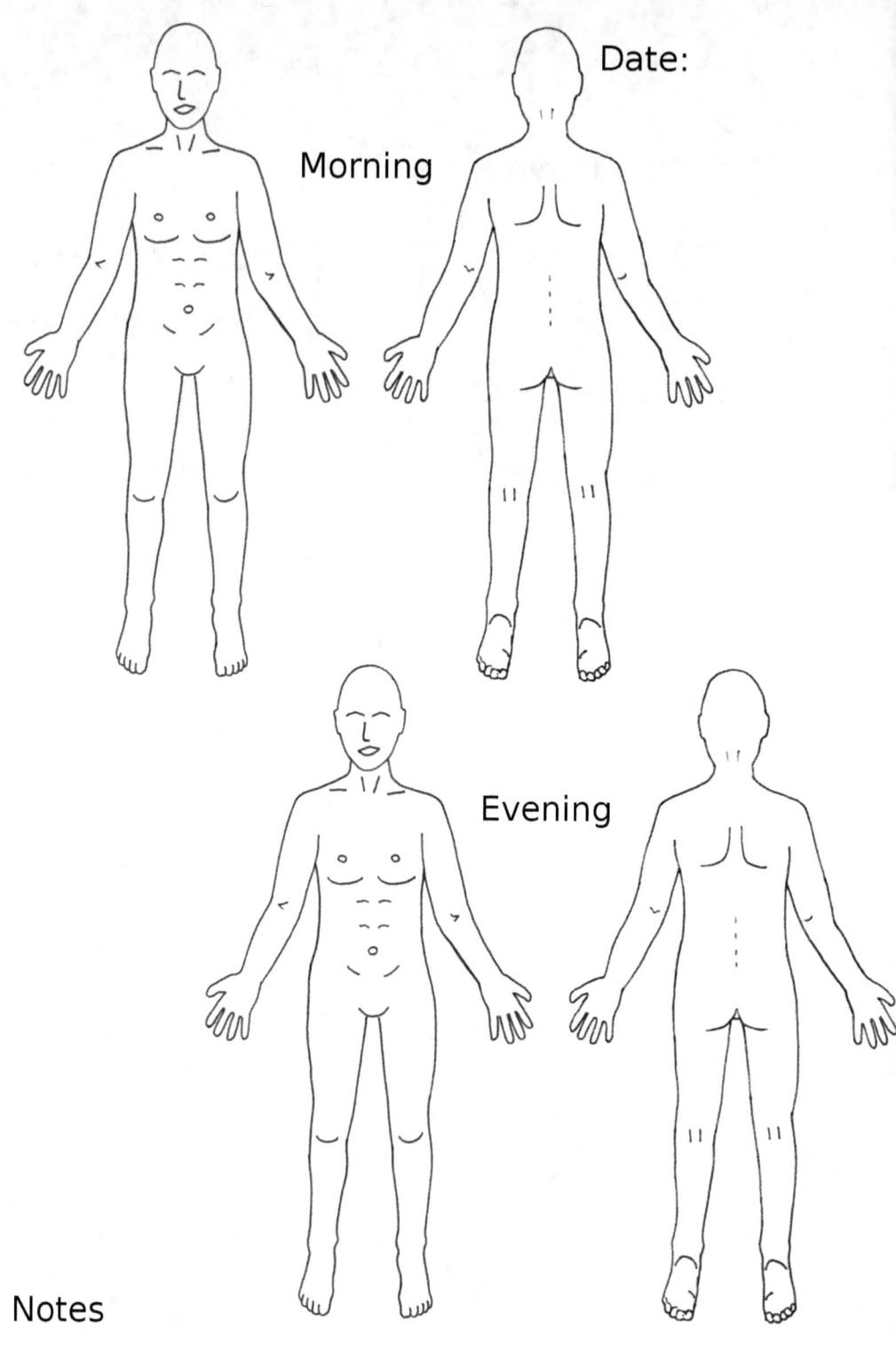

Morning

Date:

Evening

Notes

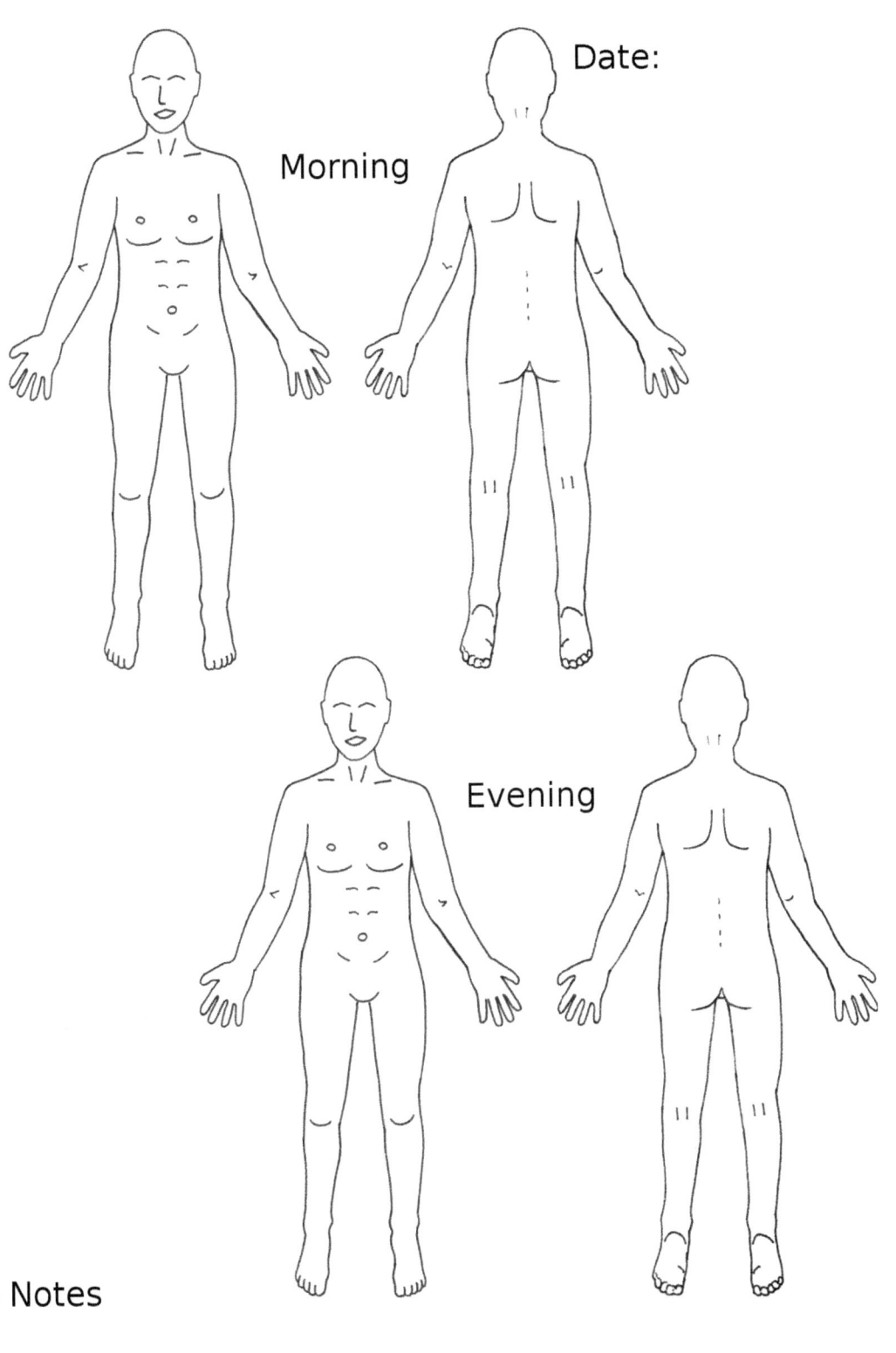

Morning

Date:

Evening

Notes

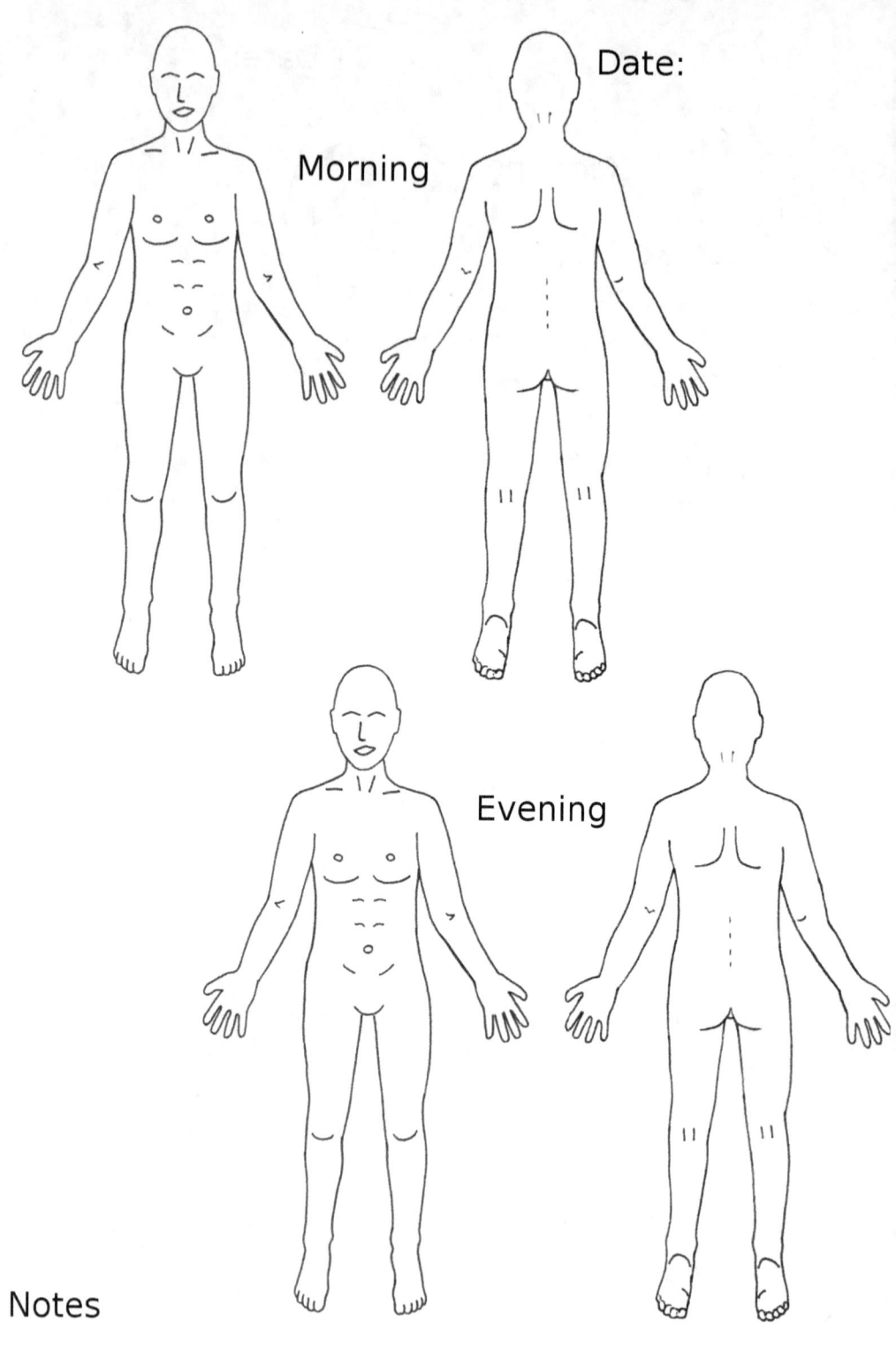

Date:

Morning

Evening

Notes

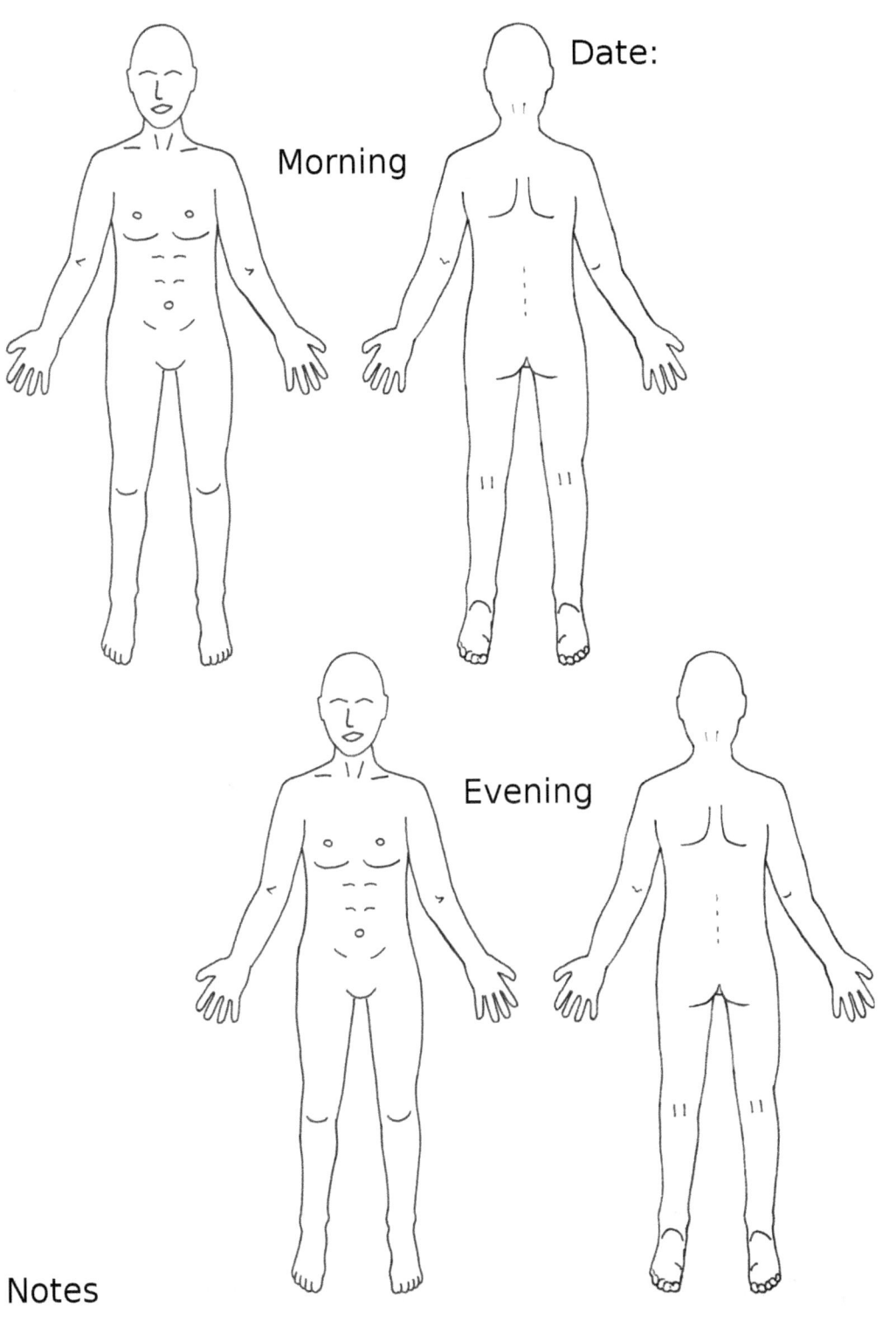

Morning

Date:

Evening

Notes

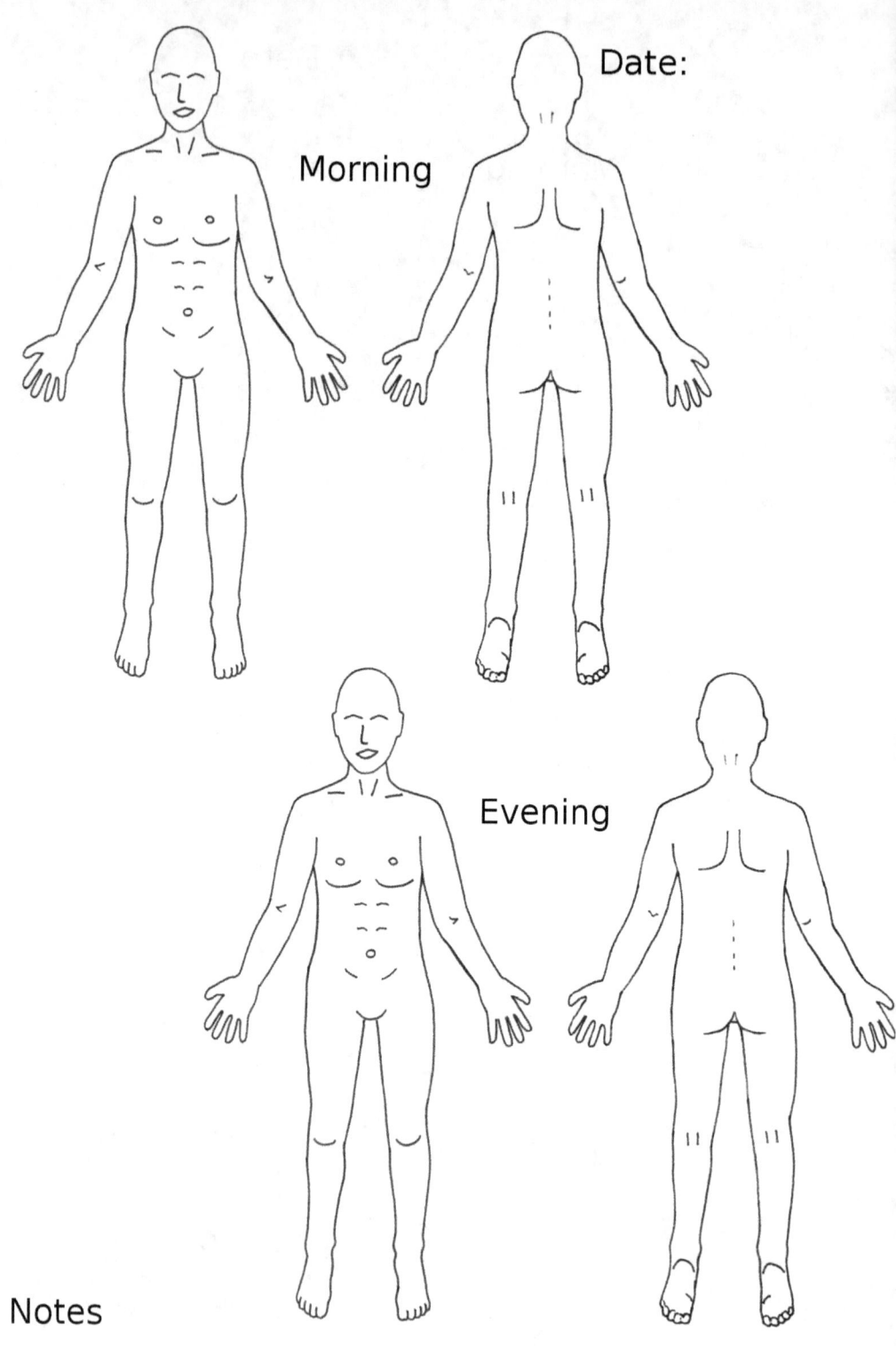

Date:

Morning

Evening

Notes

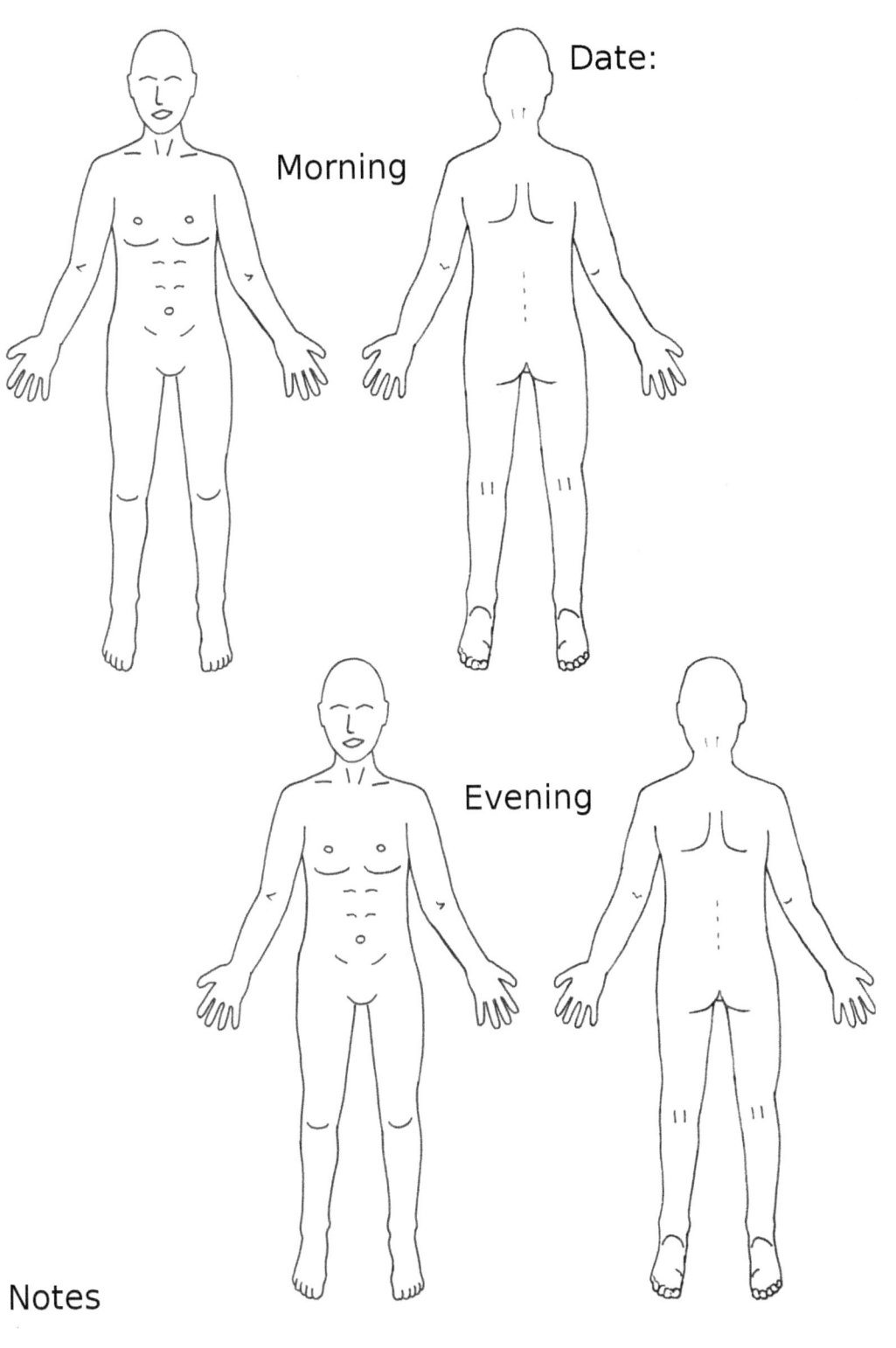

Date:

Morning

Evening

Notes

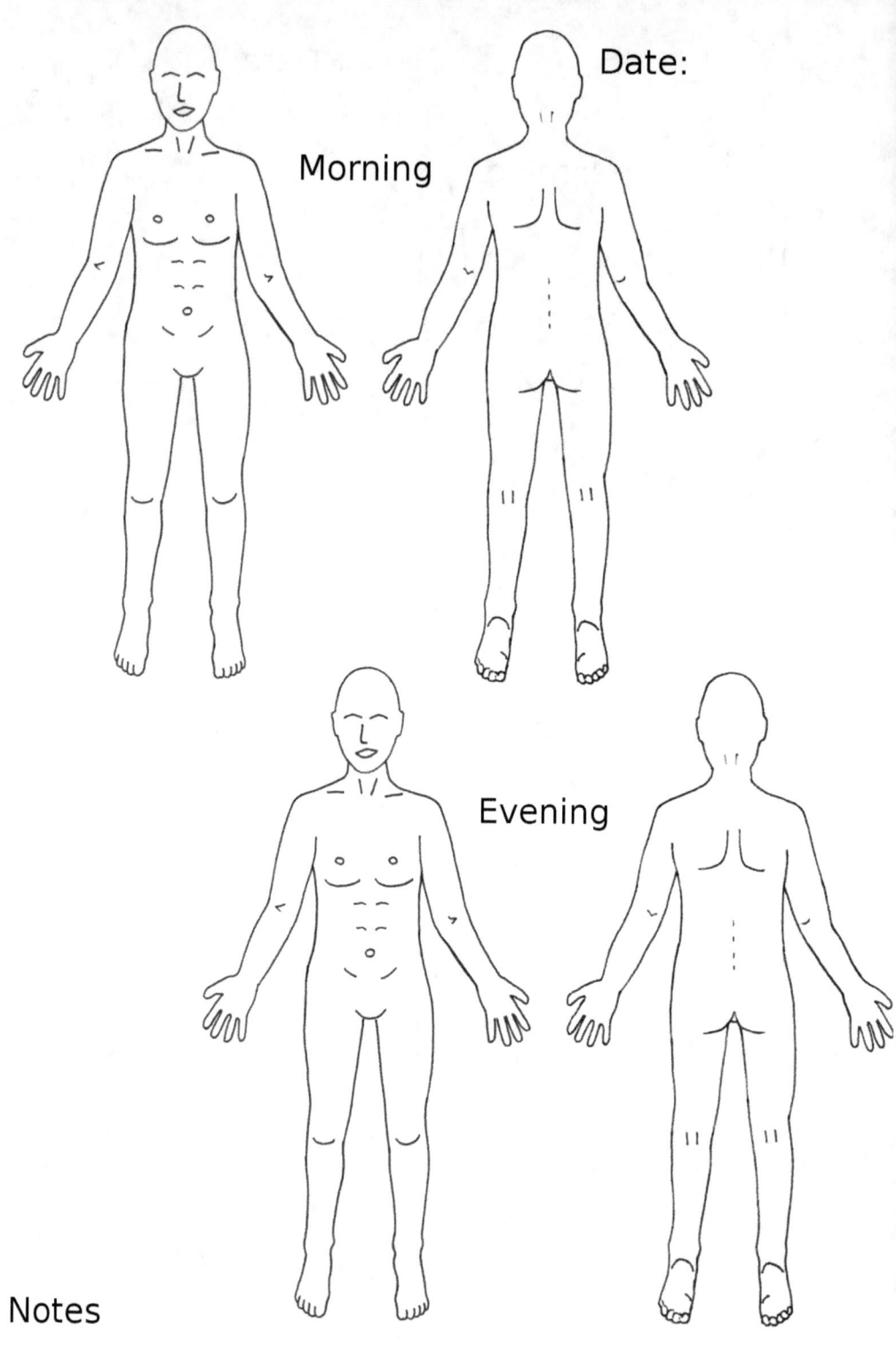

Date:

Morning

Evening

Notes

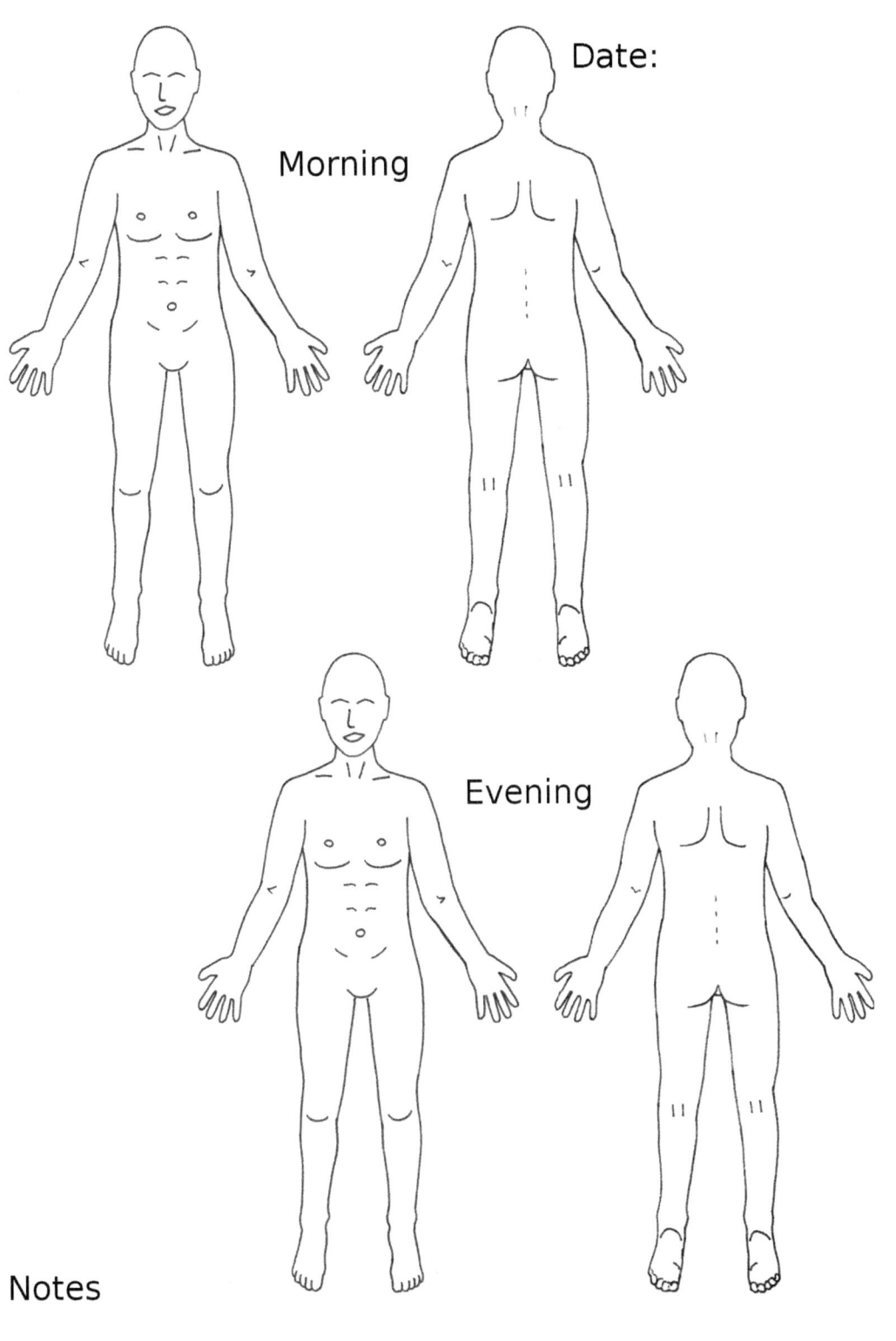

Morning

Date:

Evening

Notes

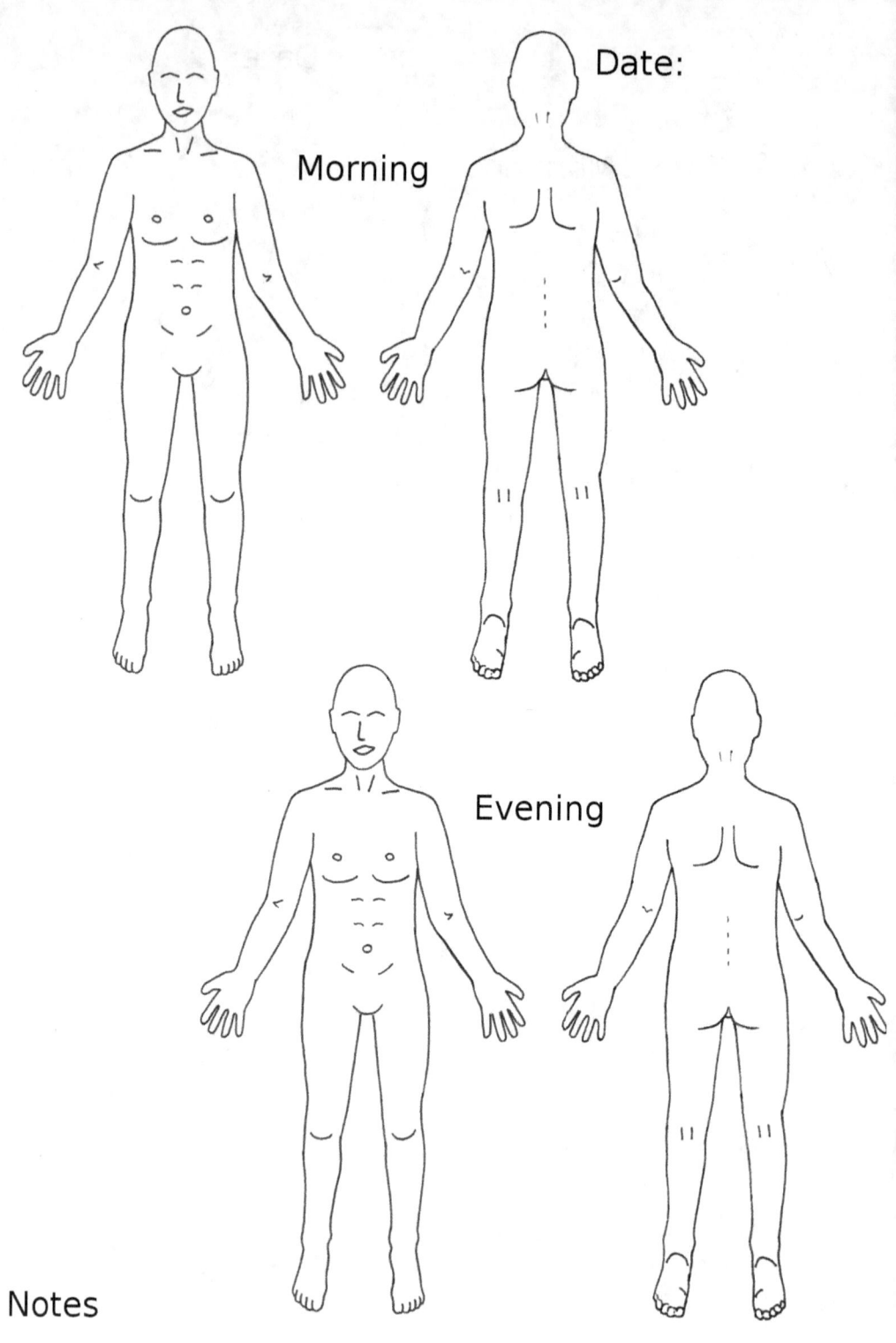

Morning

Date:

Evening

Notes

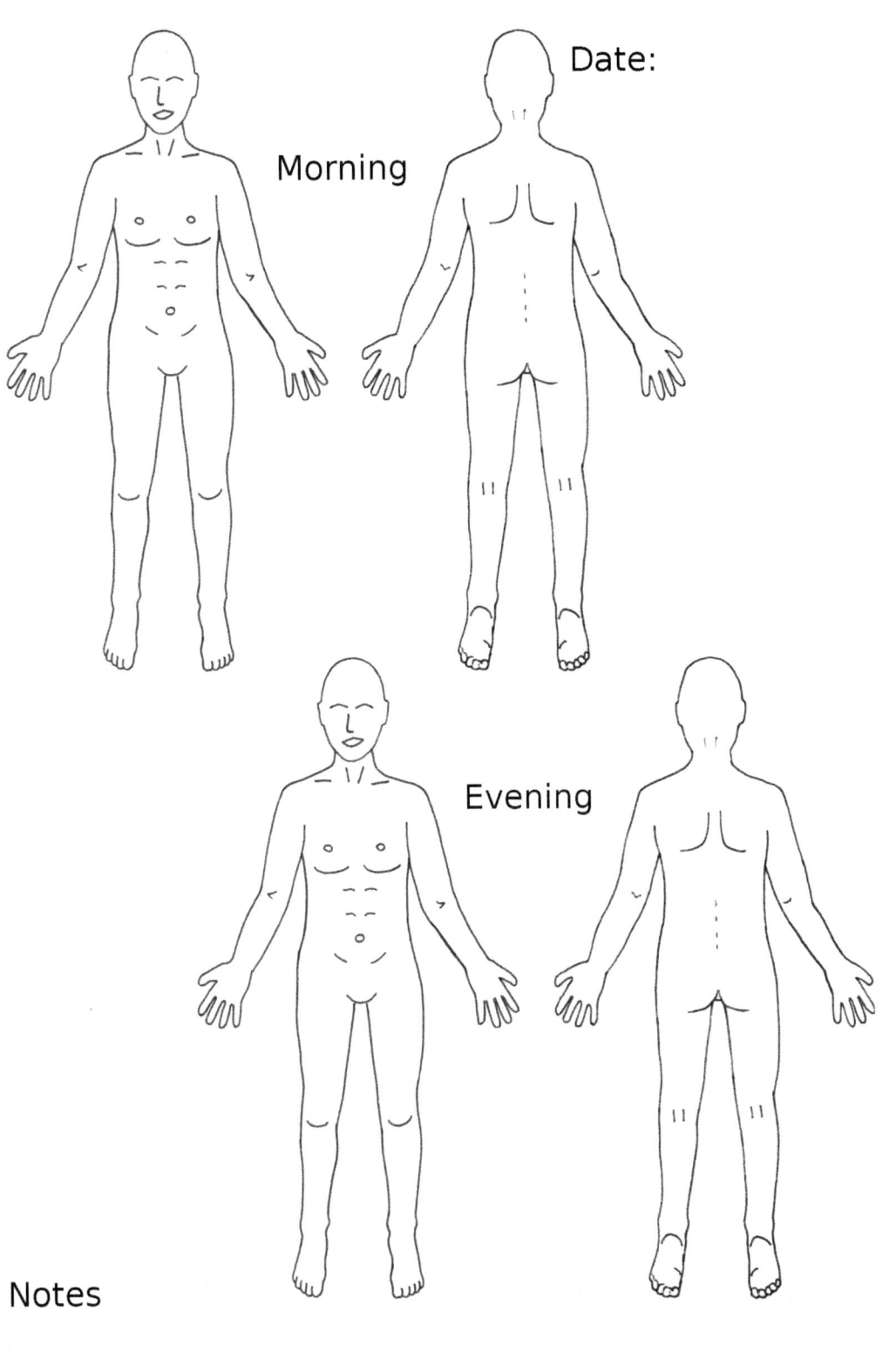

Morning

Date:

Evening

Notes

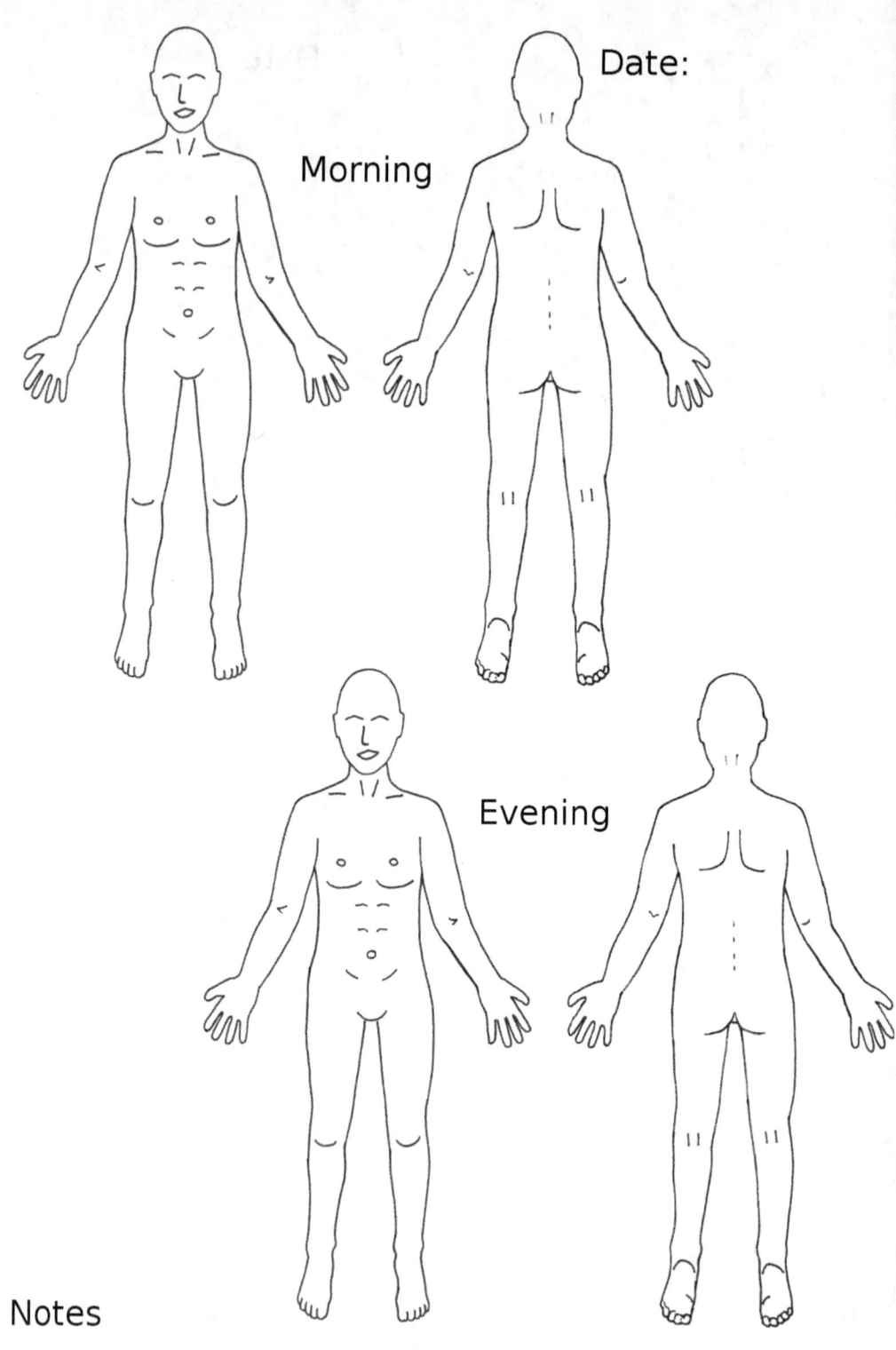

Morning

Date:

Evening

Notes

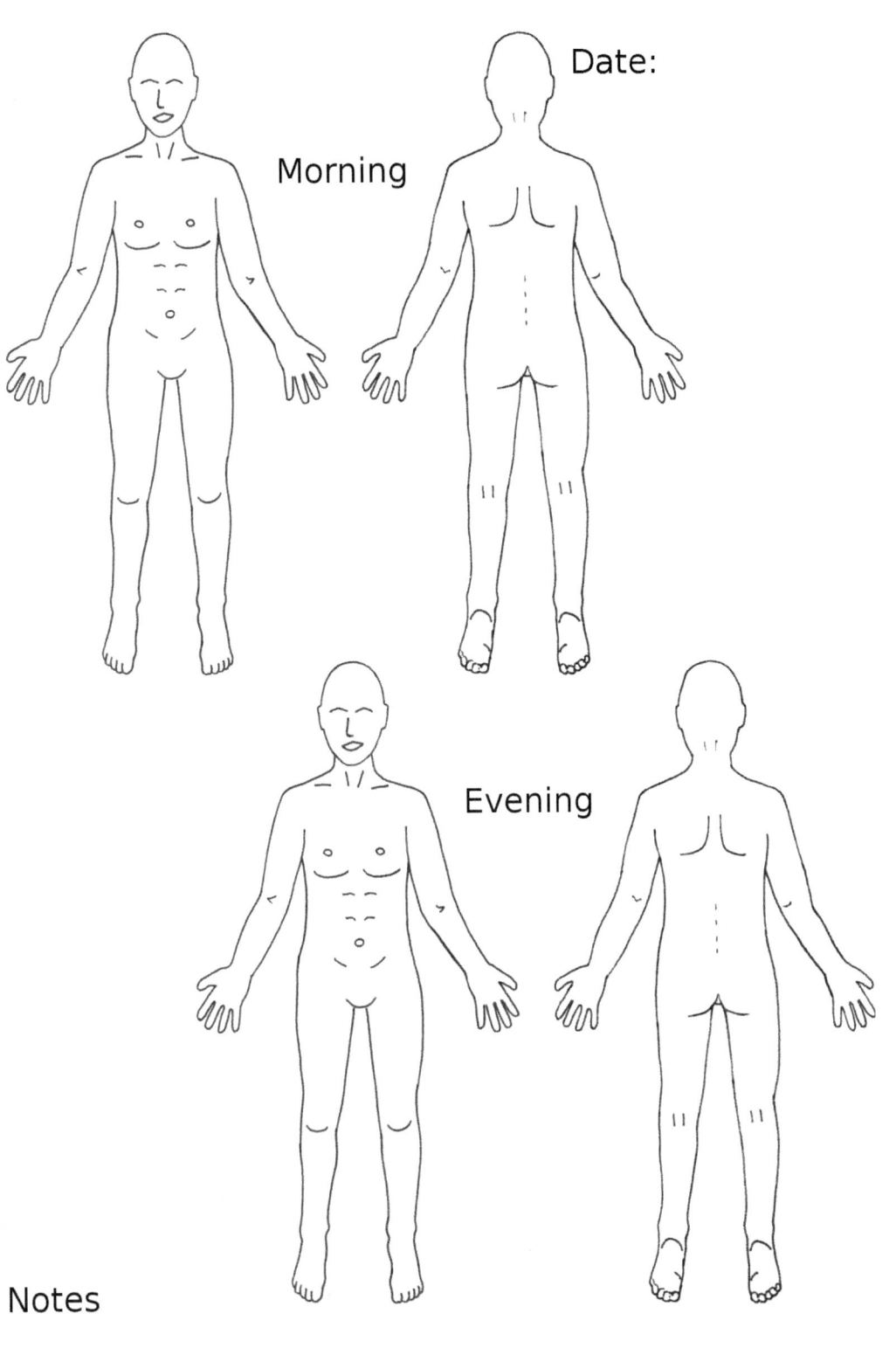

Date:

Morning

Evening

Notes

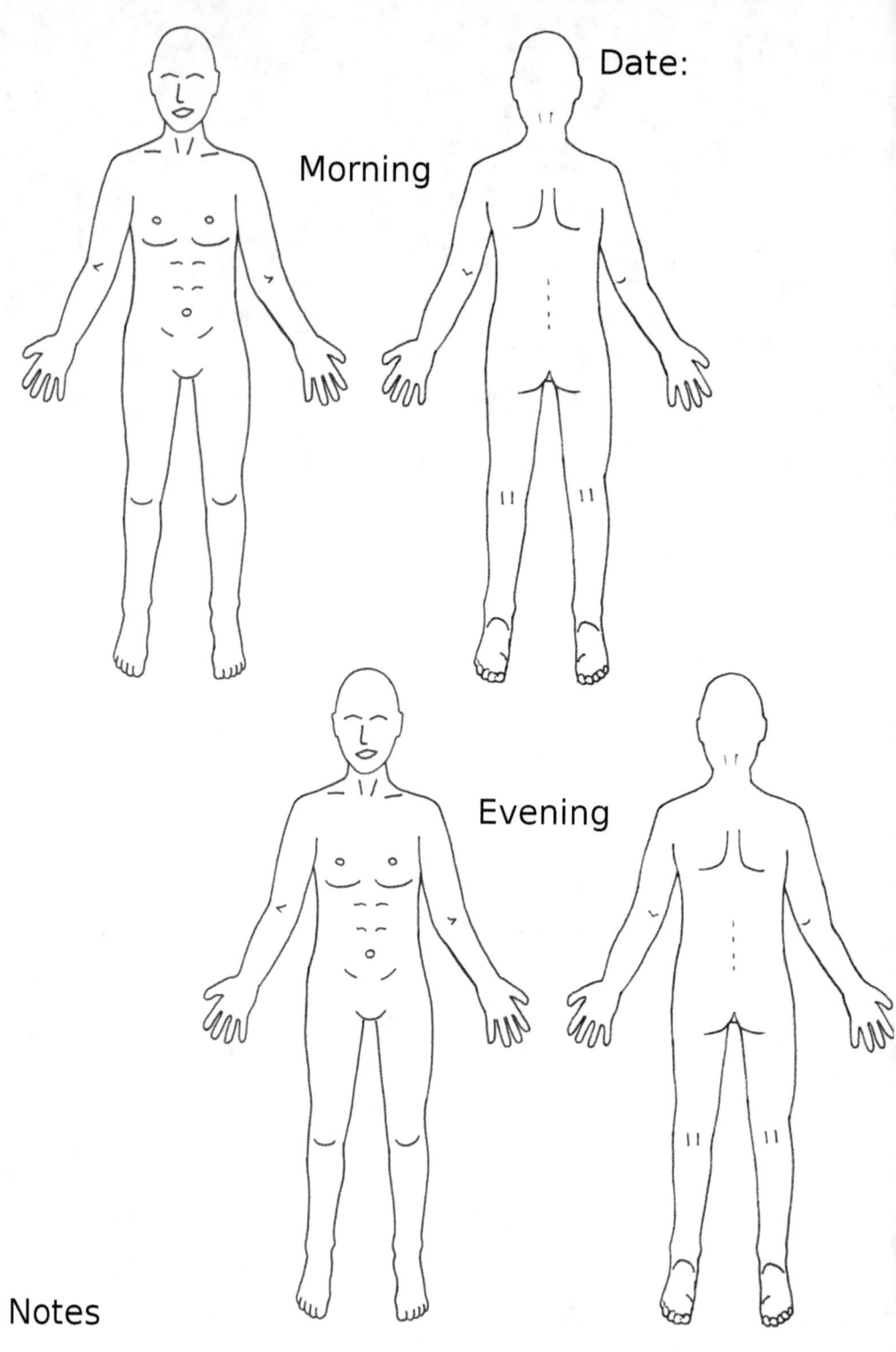

Morning

Date:

Evening

Notes

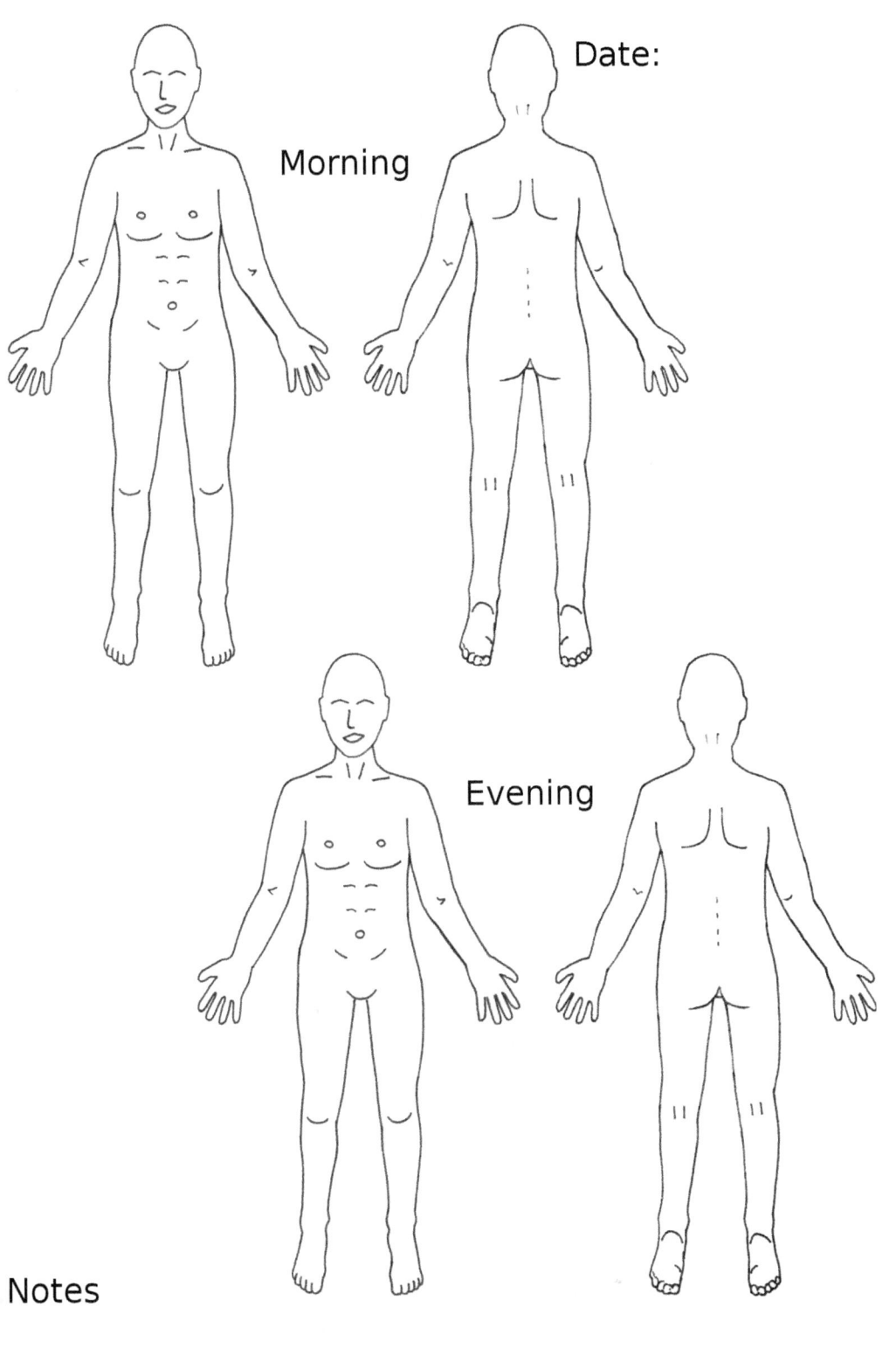

Morning

Date:

Evening

Notes

Date:

Morning

Evening

Notes

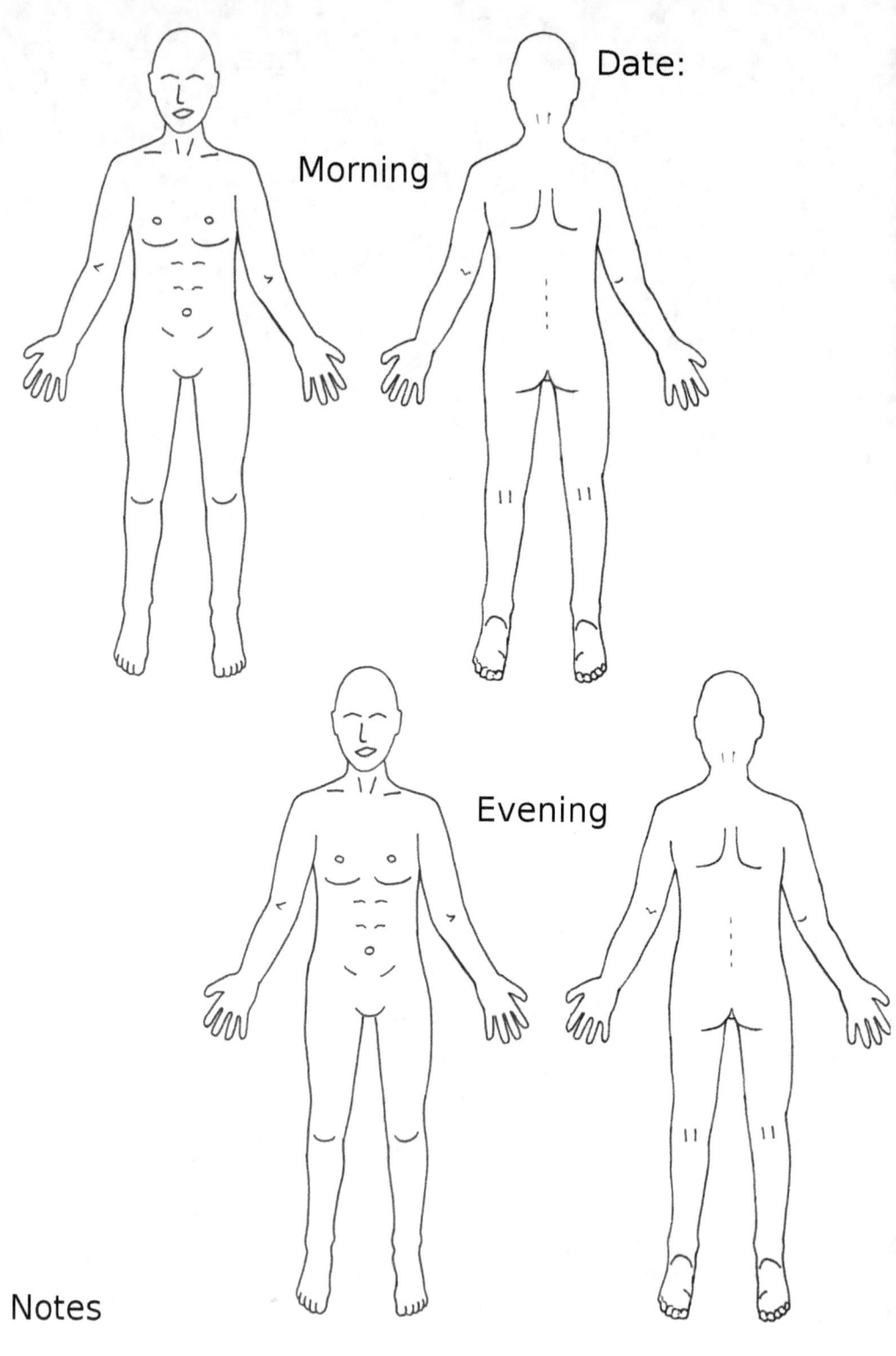

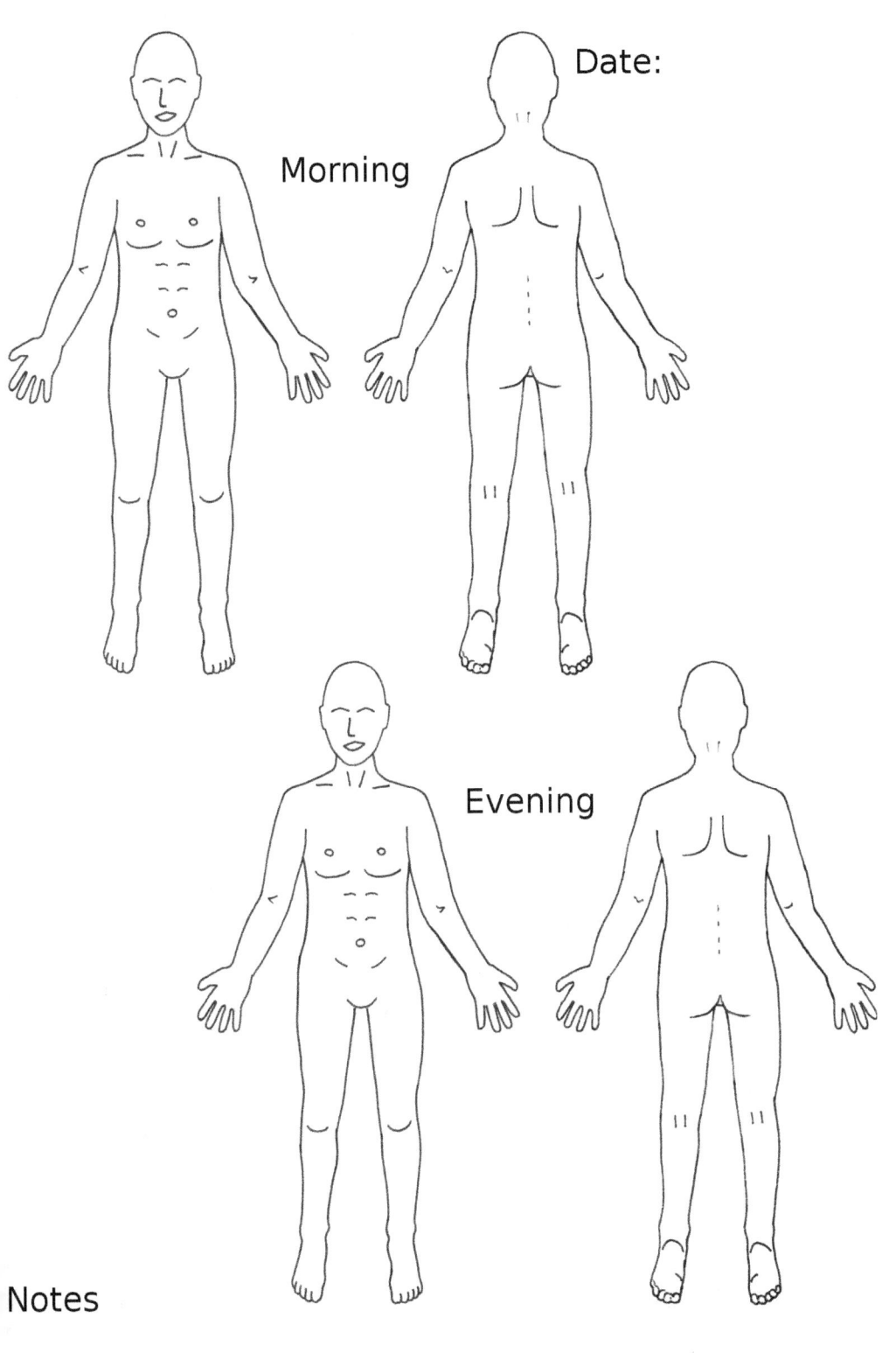

Morning

Date:

Evening

Notes

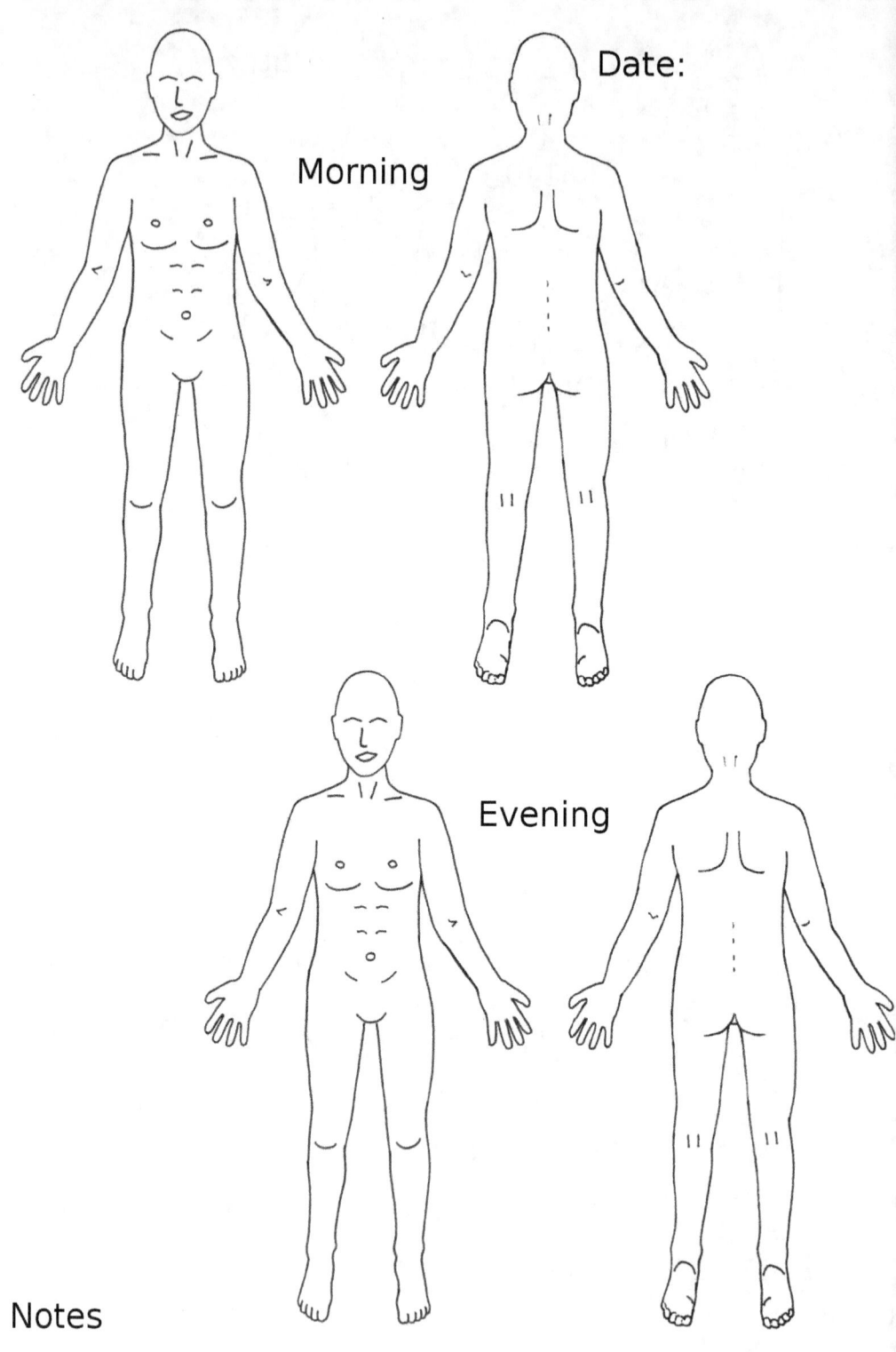

Date:

Morning

Evening

Notes

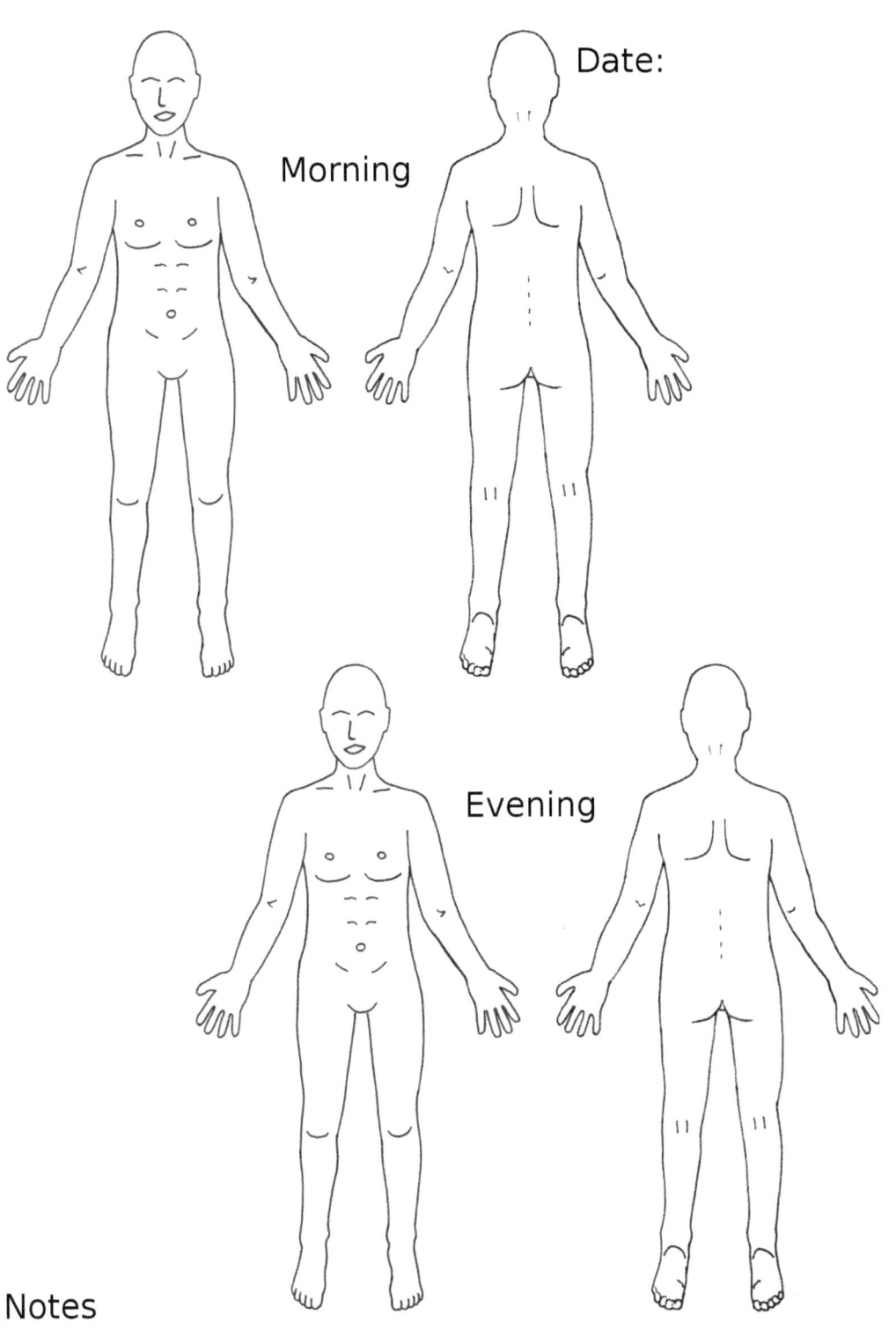

Date:

Morning

Evening

Notes

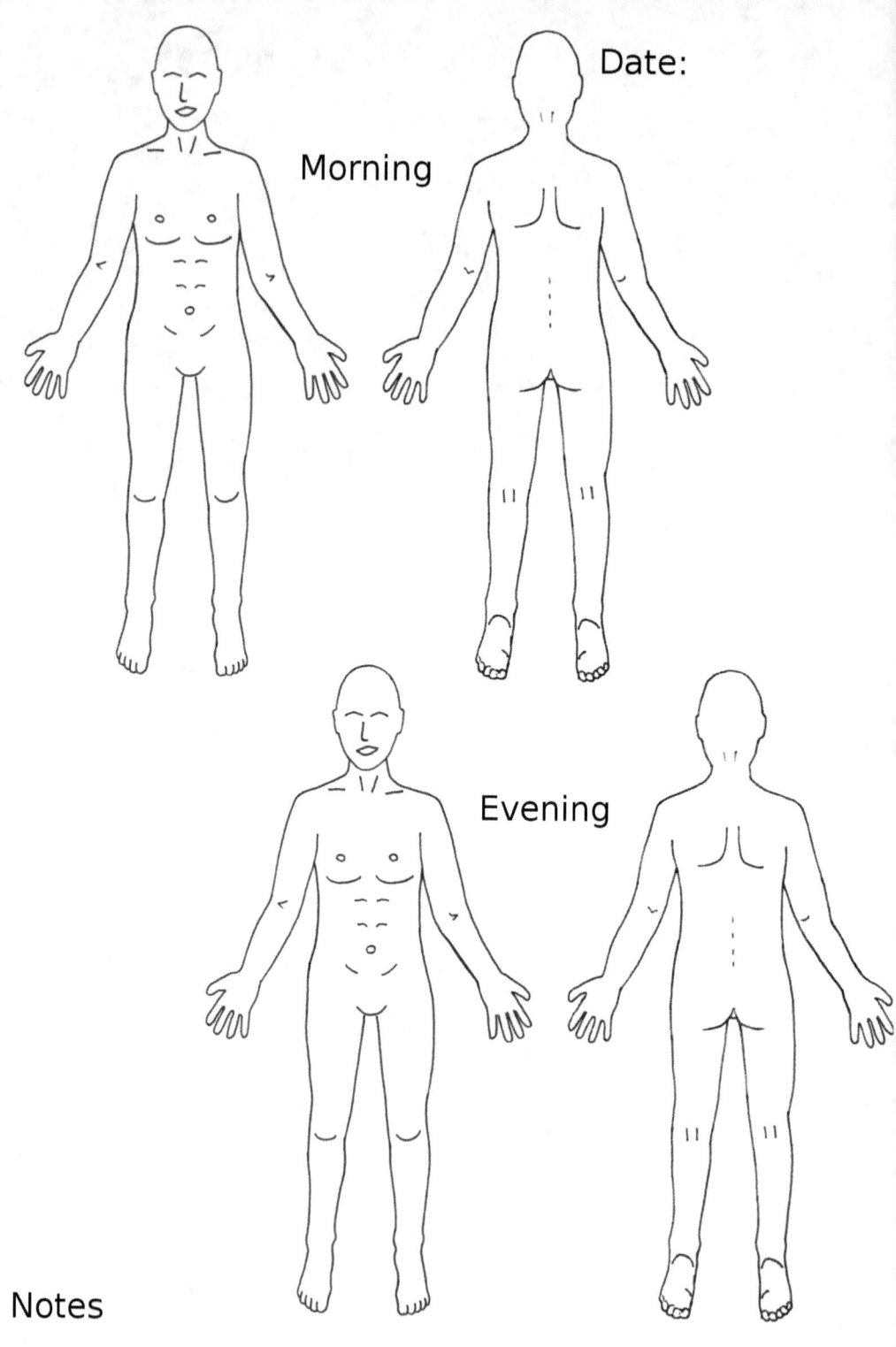

Date:

Morning

Evening

Notes

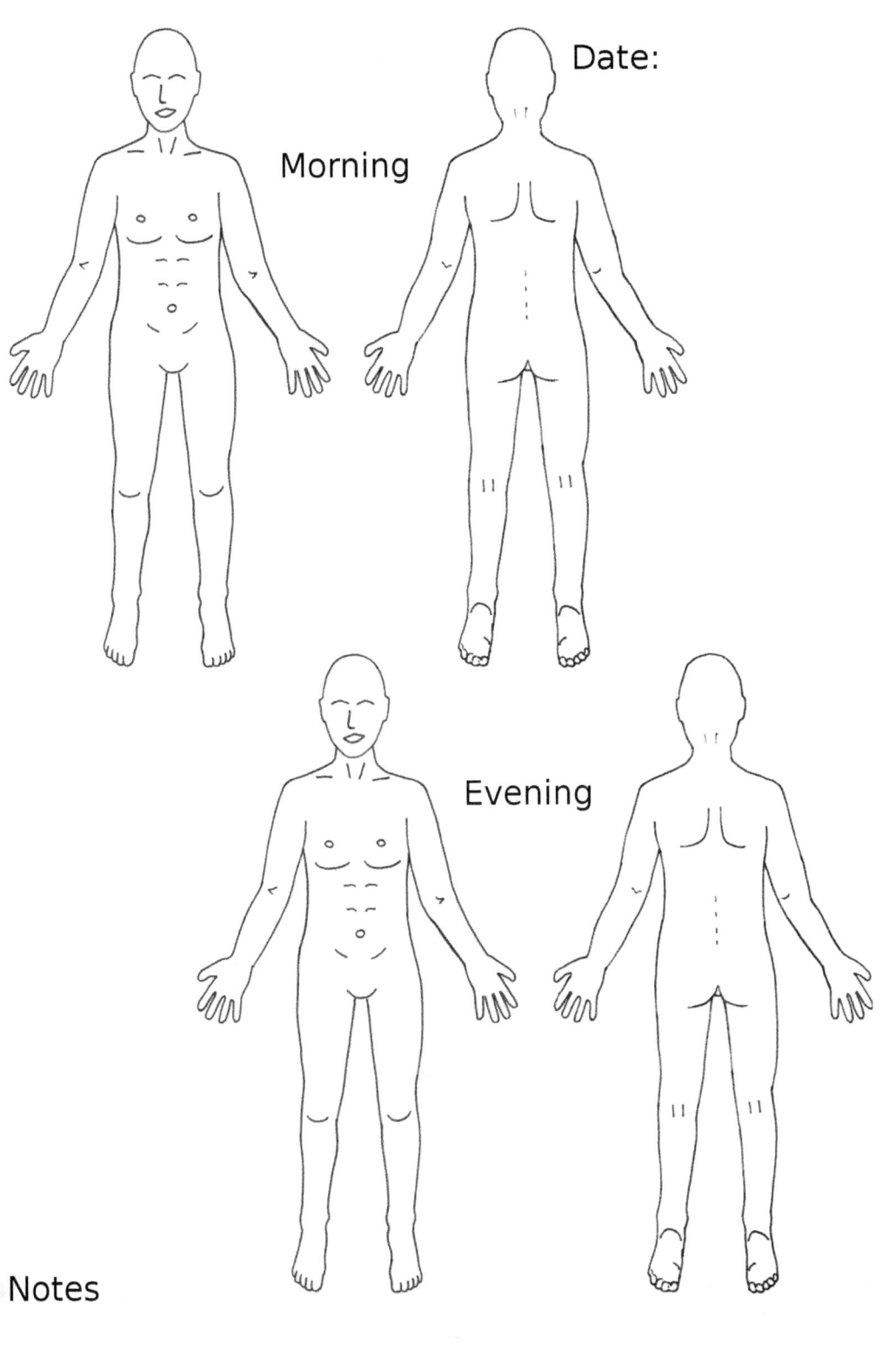

Date:

Morning

Evening

Notes

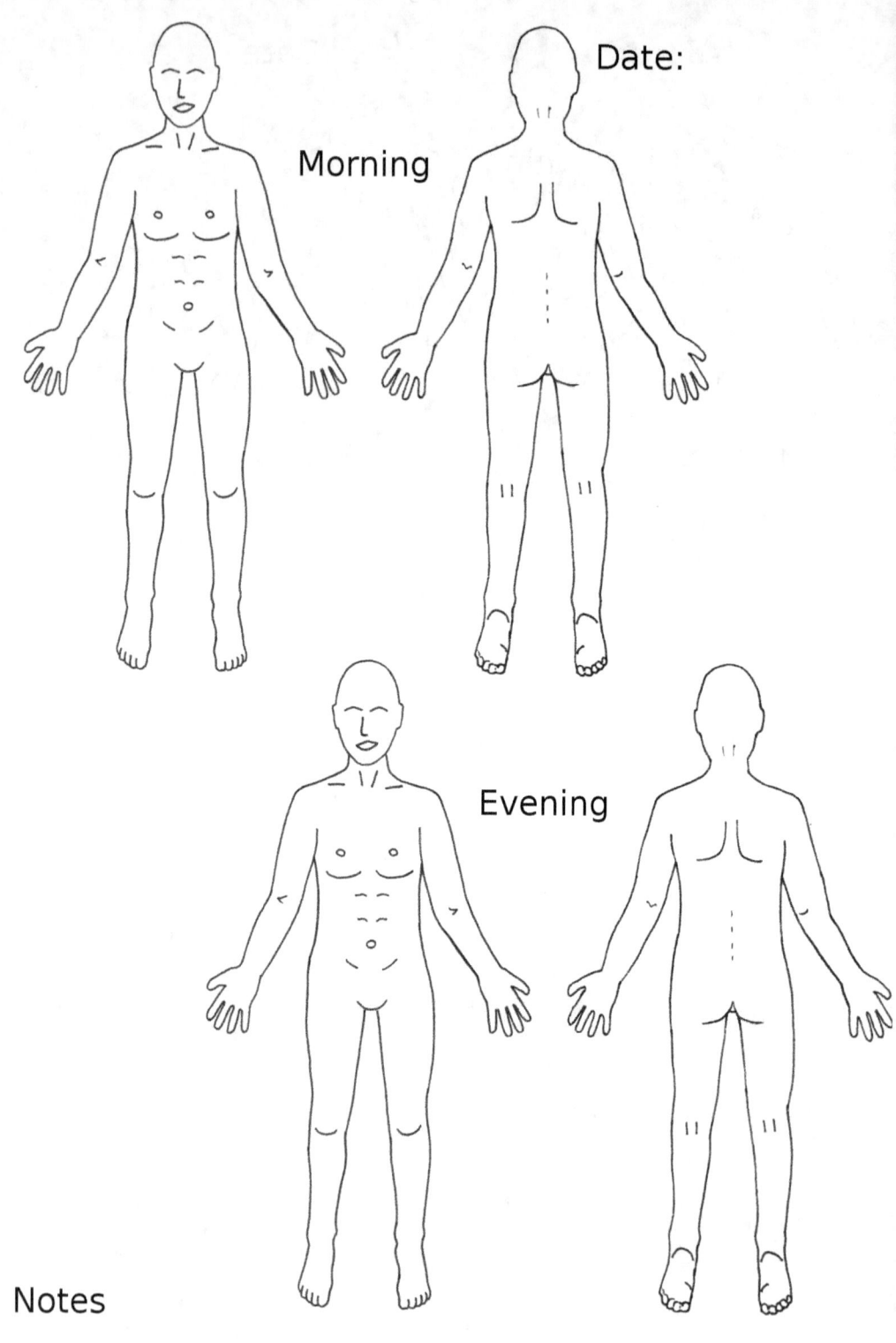

Morning

Date:

Evening

Notes

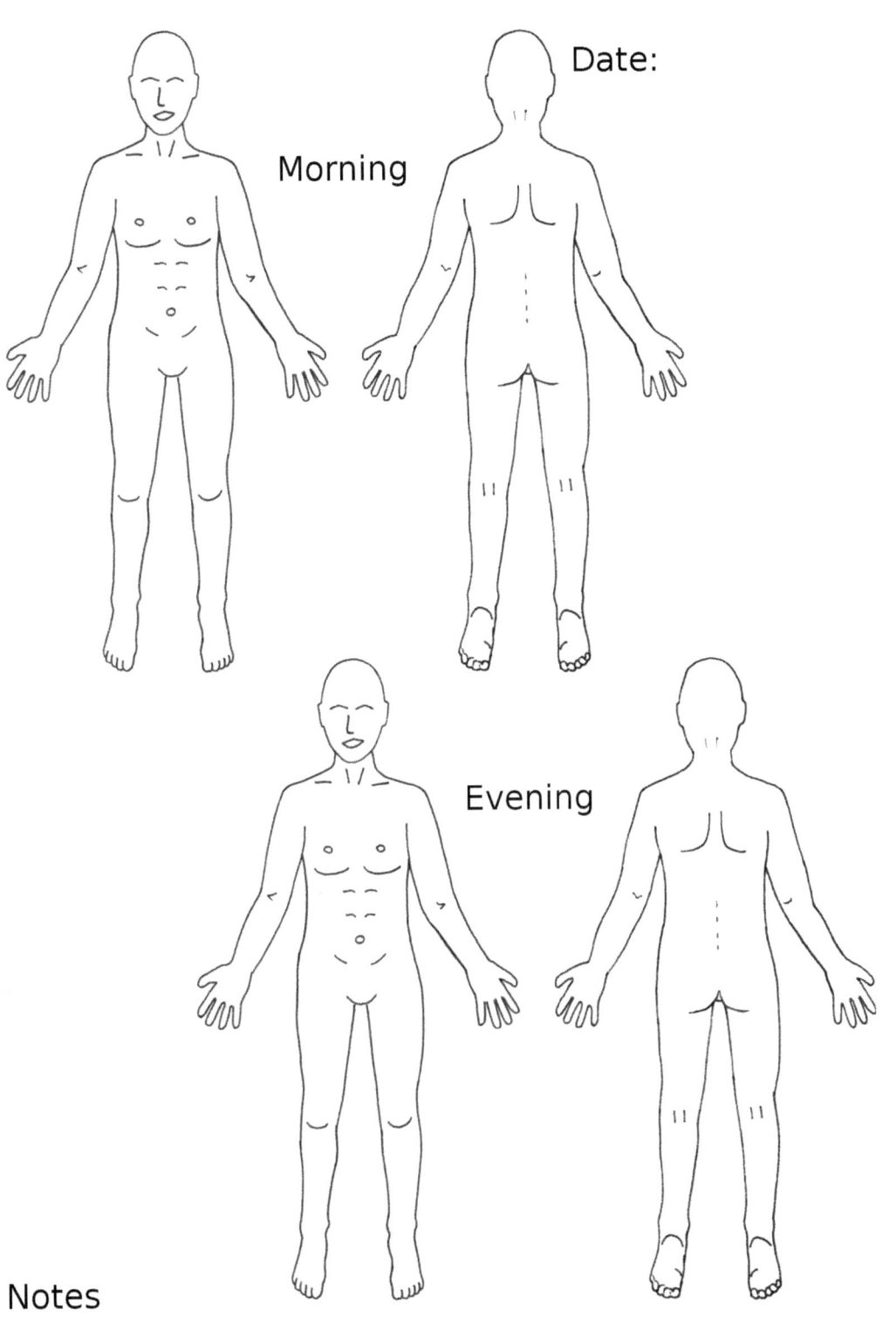

Morning

Date:

Evening

Notes

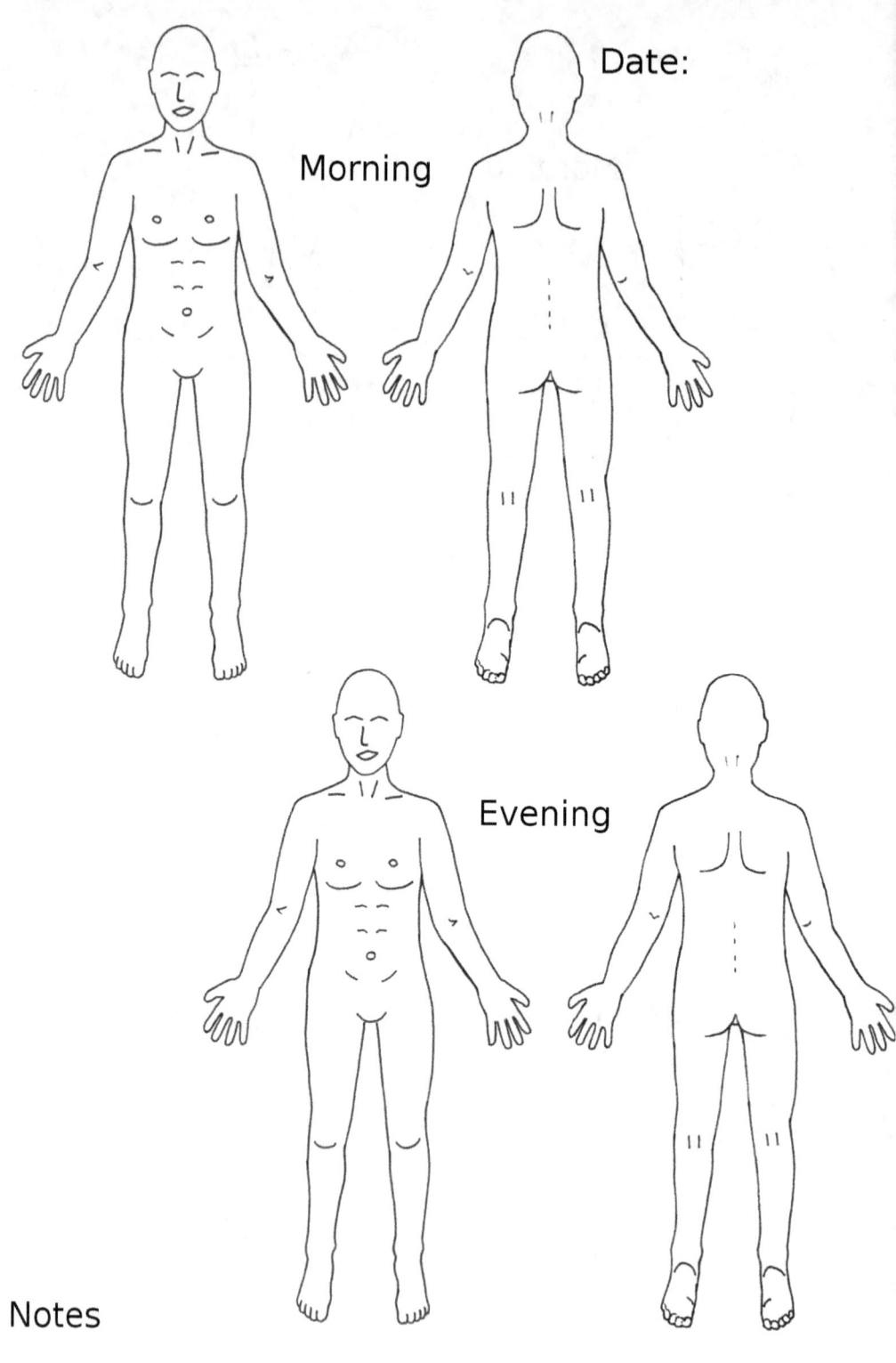

Date:

Morning

Evening

Notes

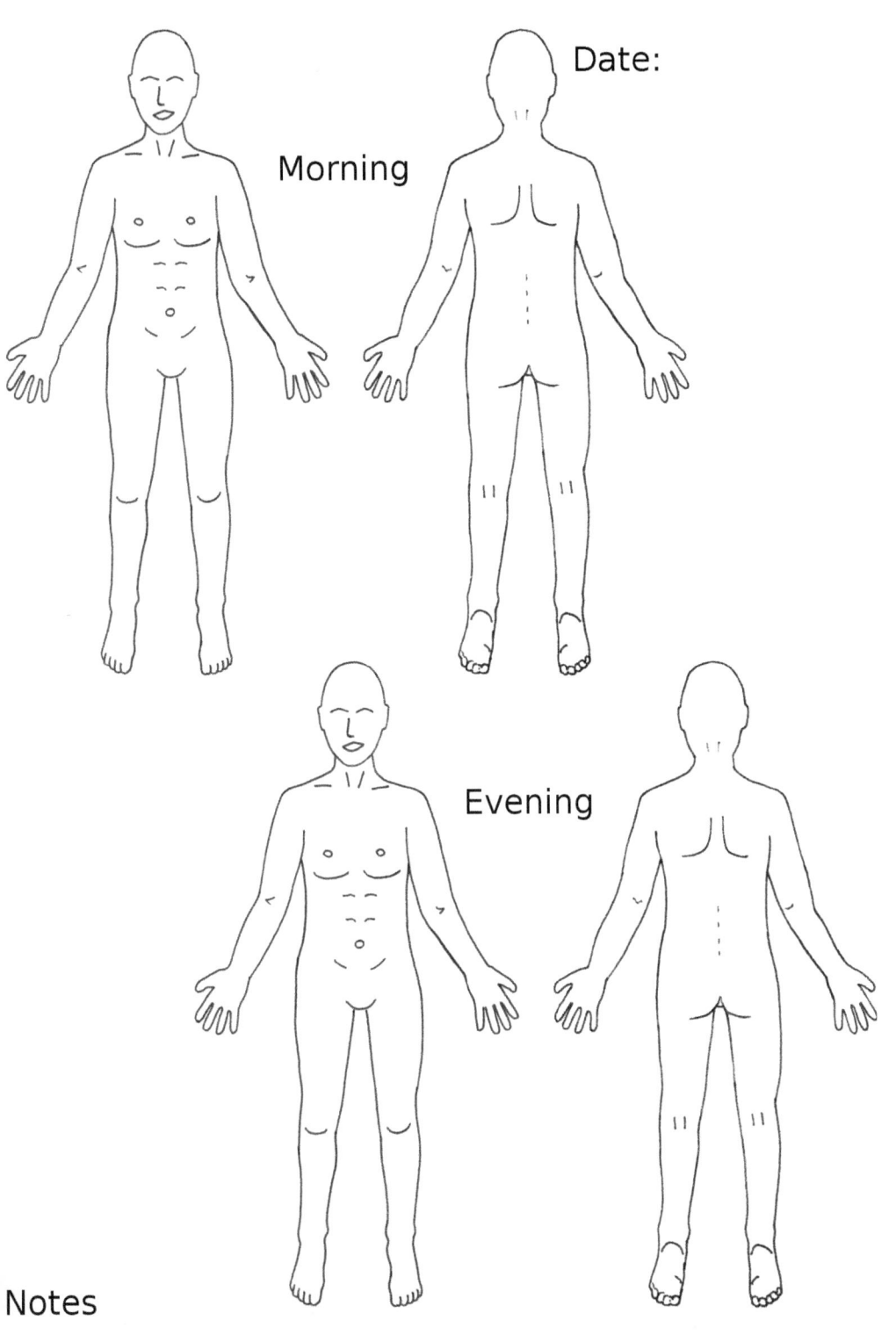

Date:

Morning

Evening

Notes

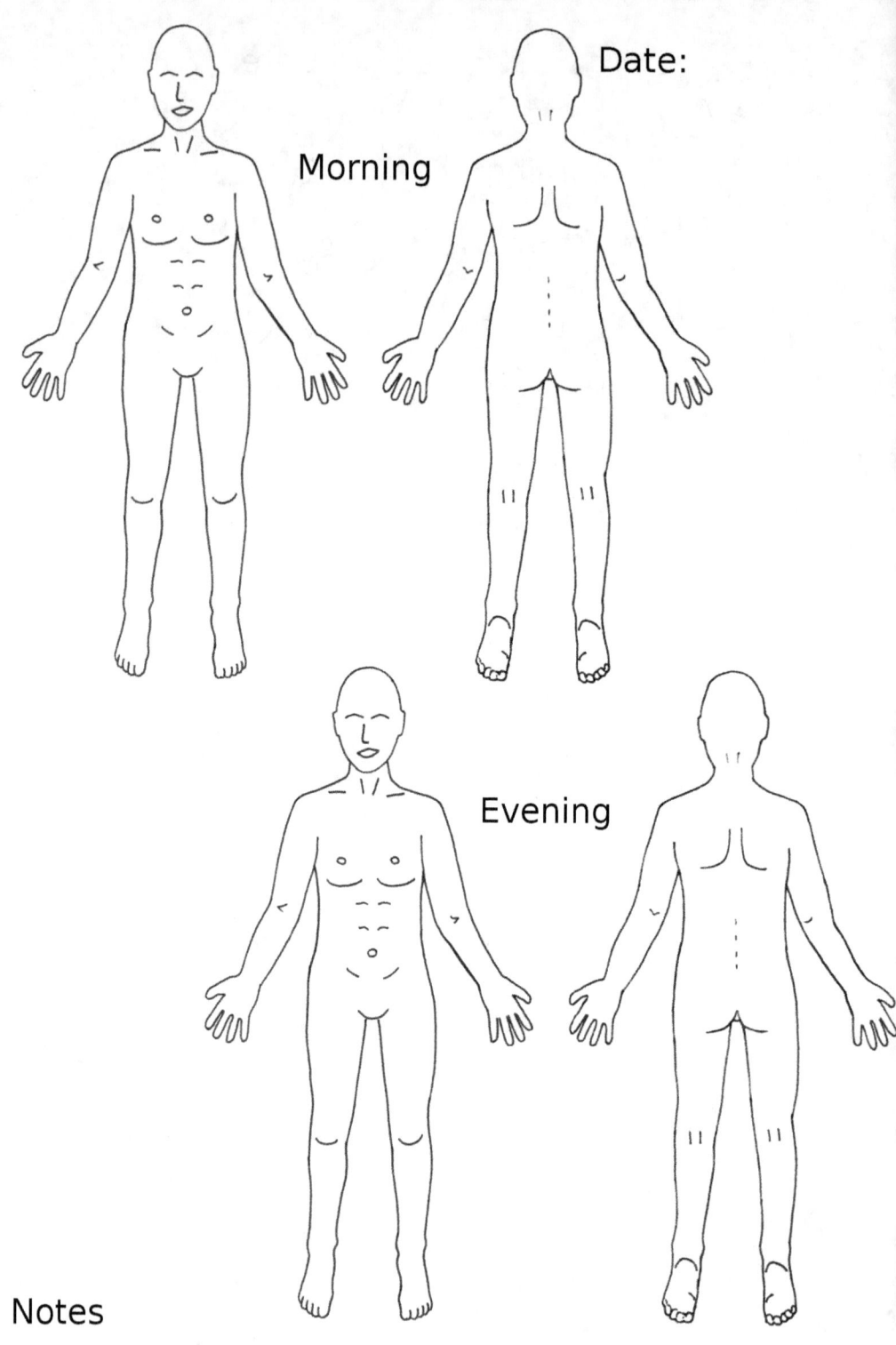

Date:

Morning

Evening

Notes

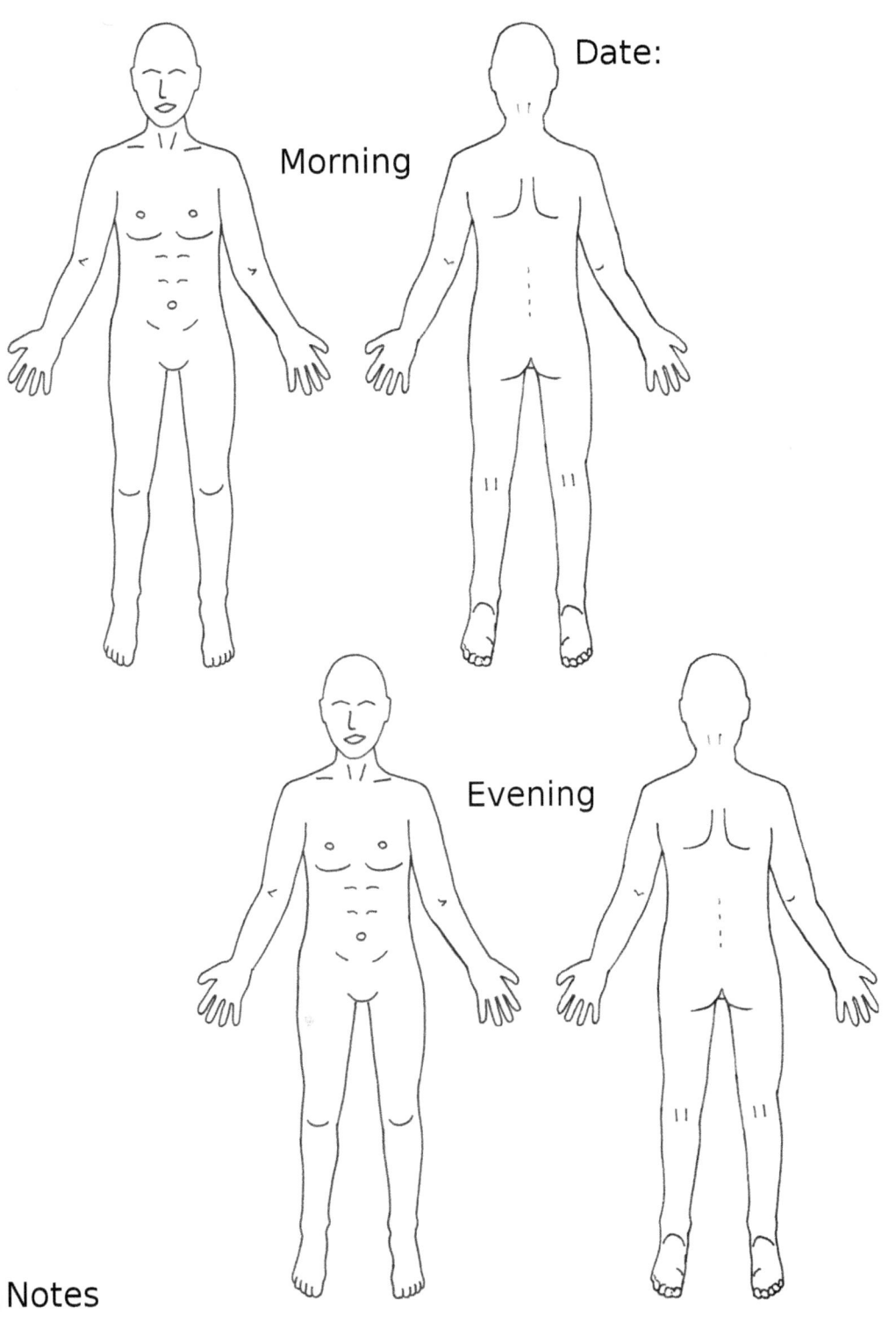

Morning

Date:

Evening

Notes

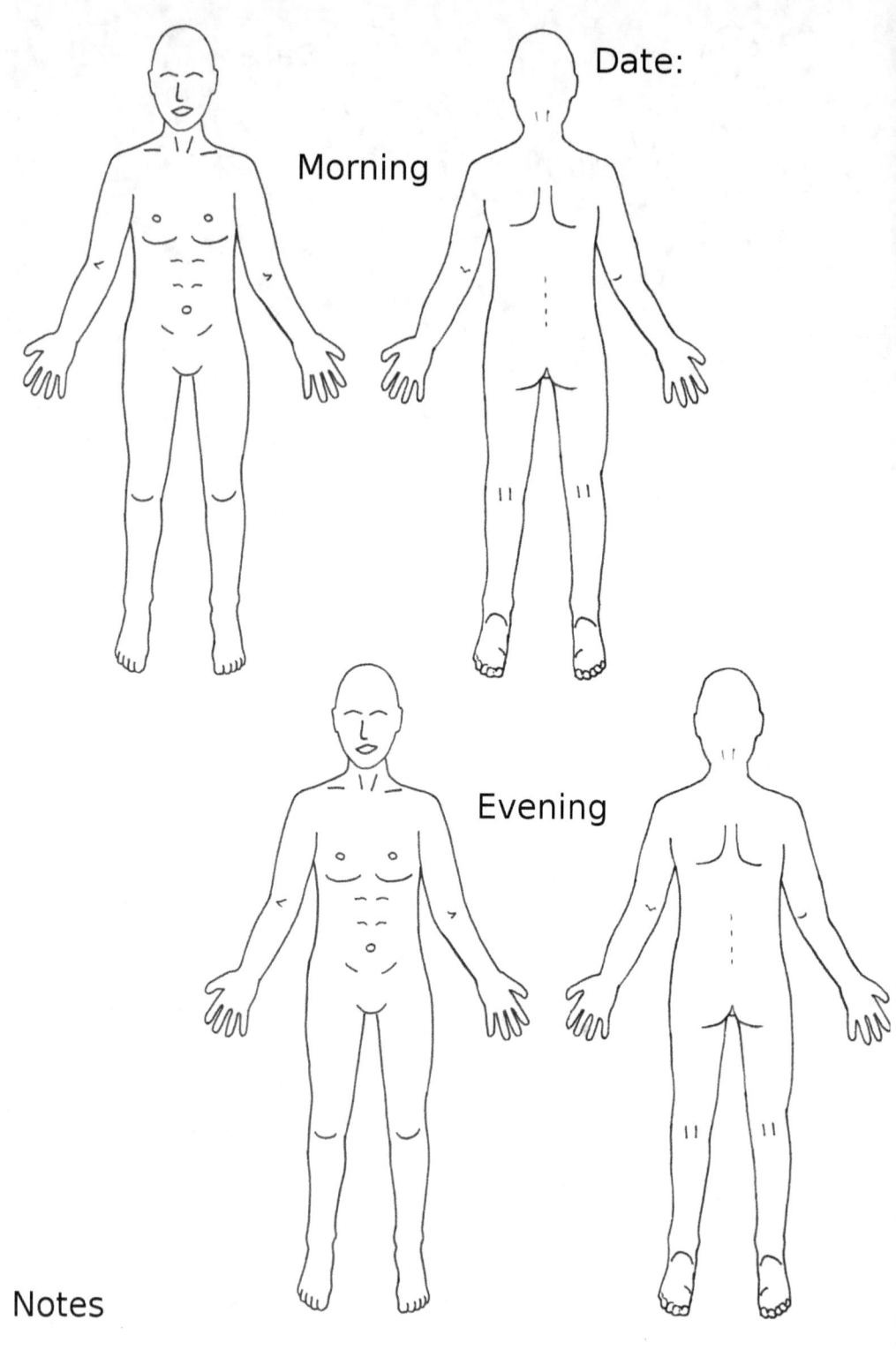

Morning

Date:

Evening

Notes

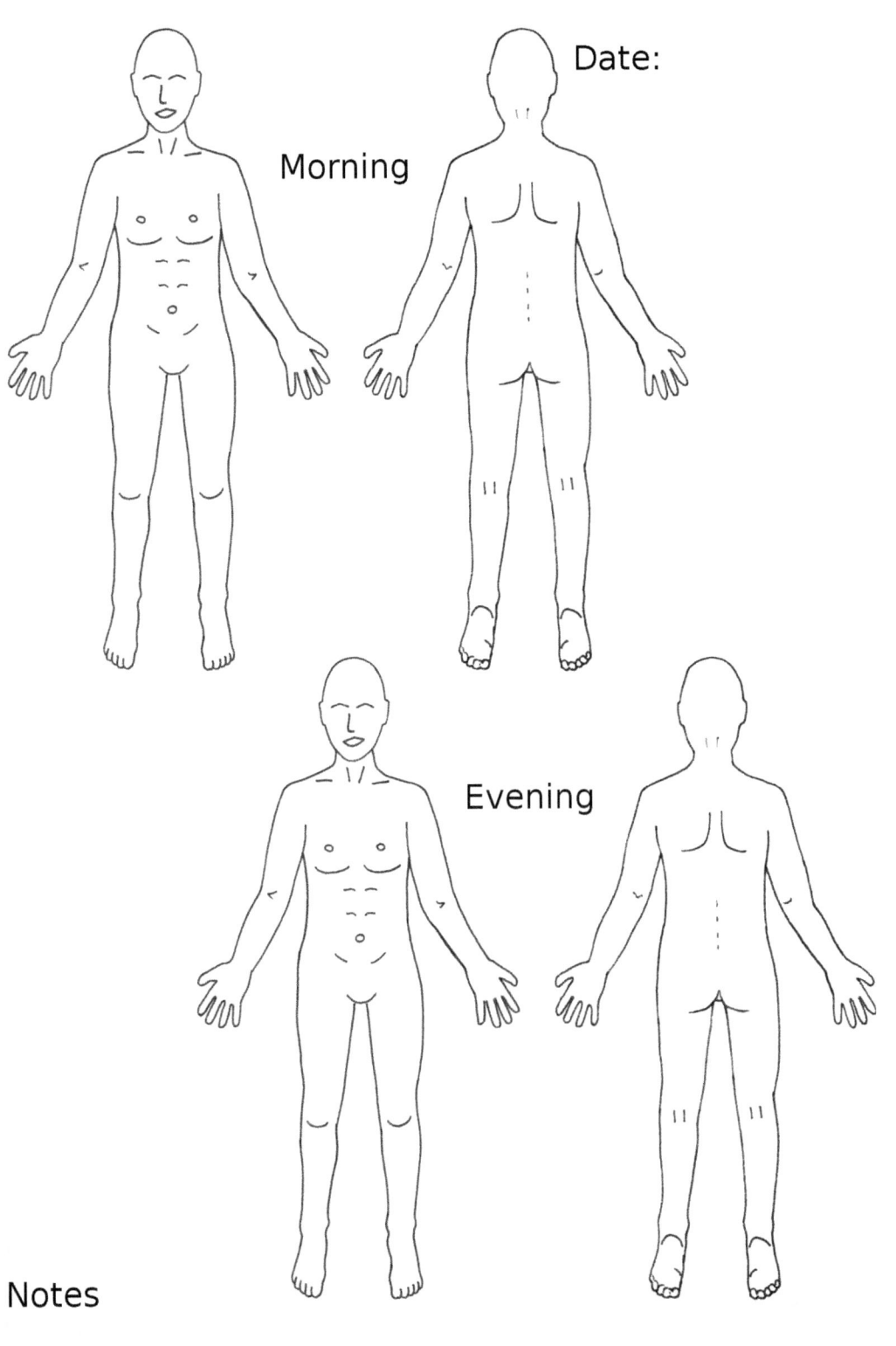

Date:

Morning

Evening

Notes

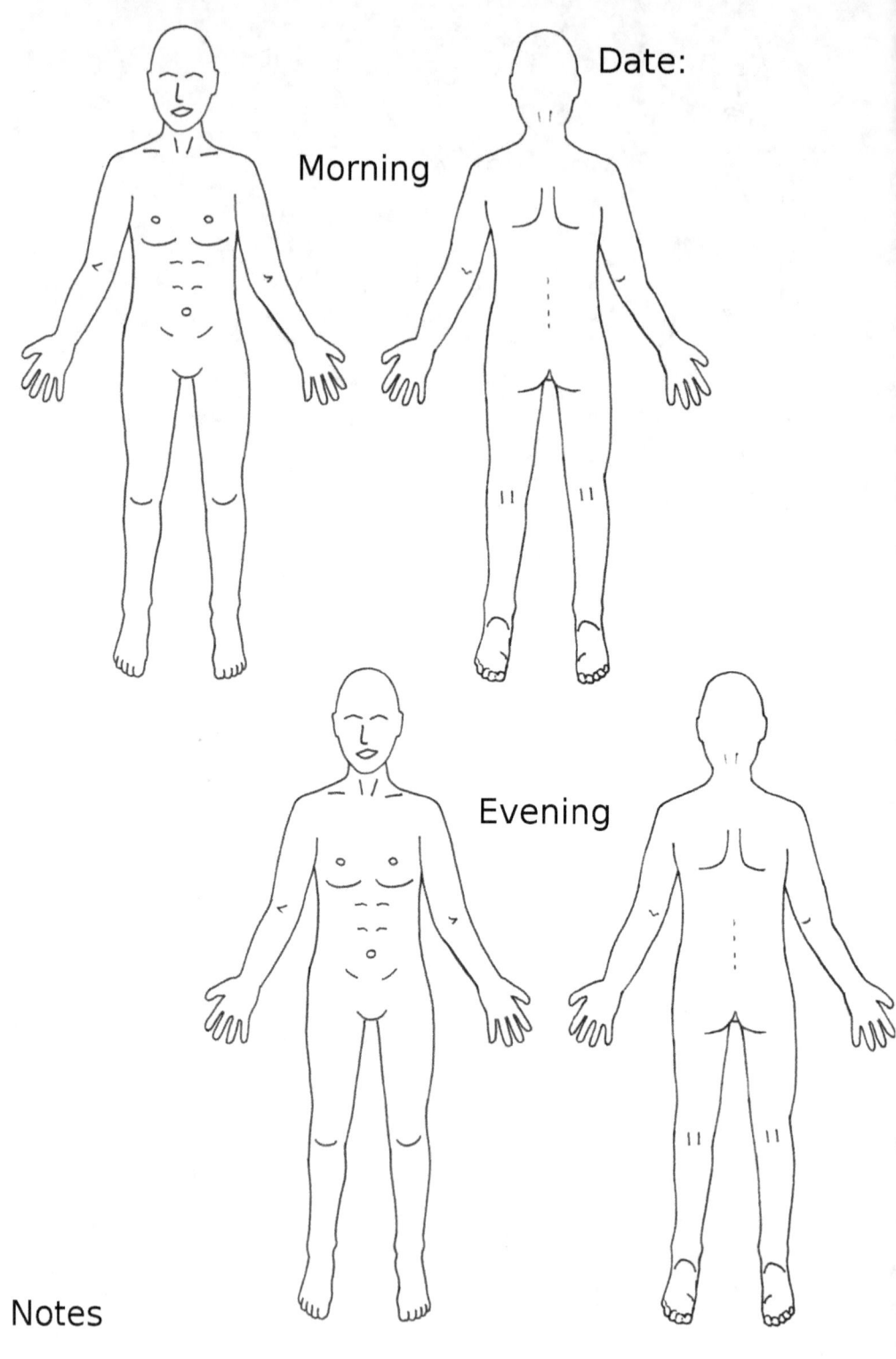

Morning

Date:

Evening

Notes

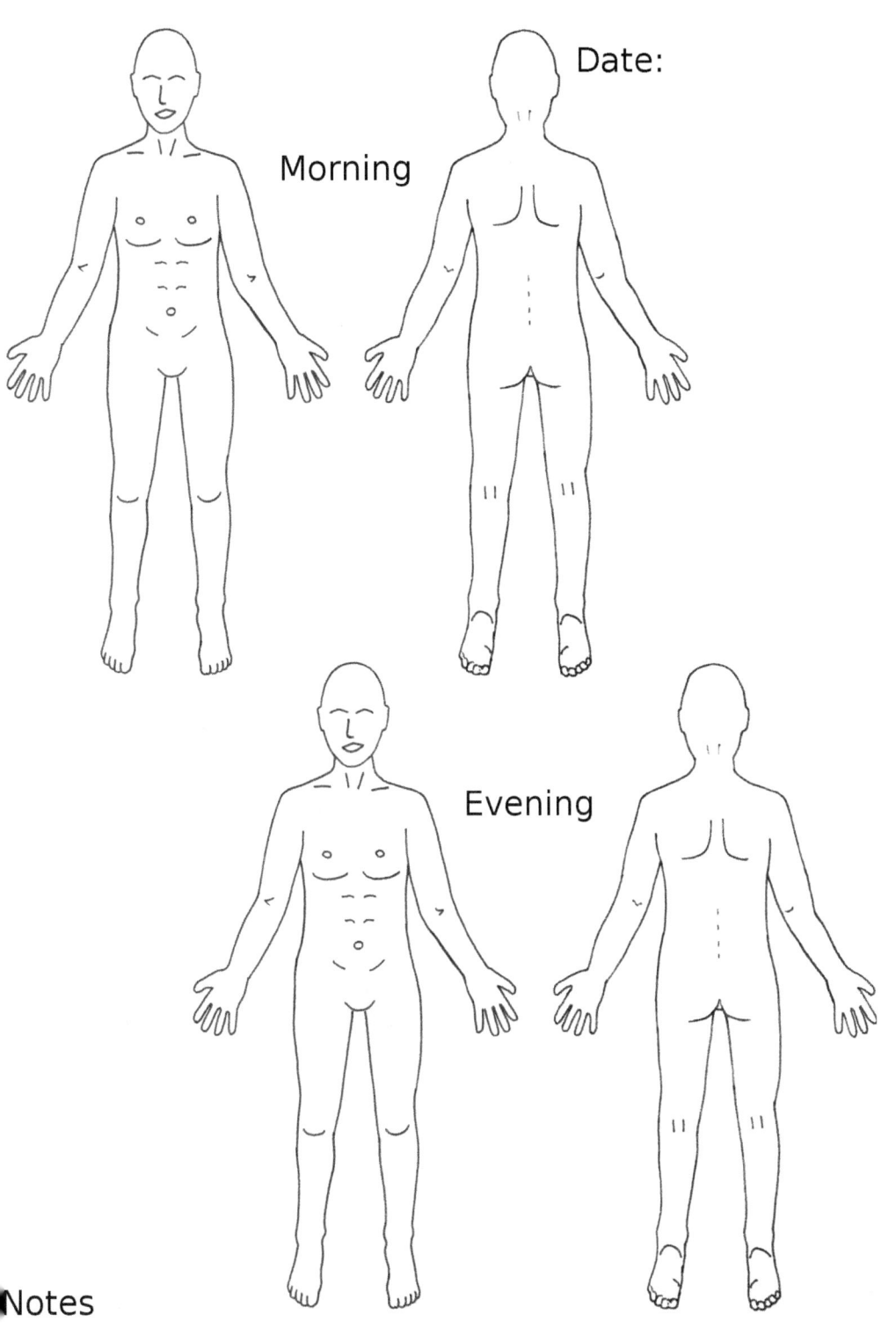

Morning

Date:

Evening

Notes

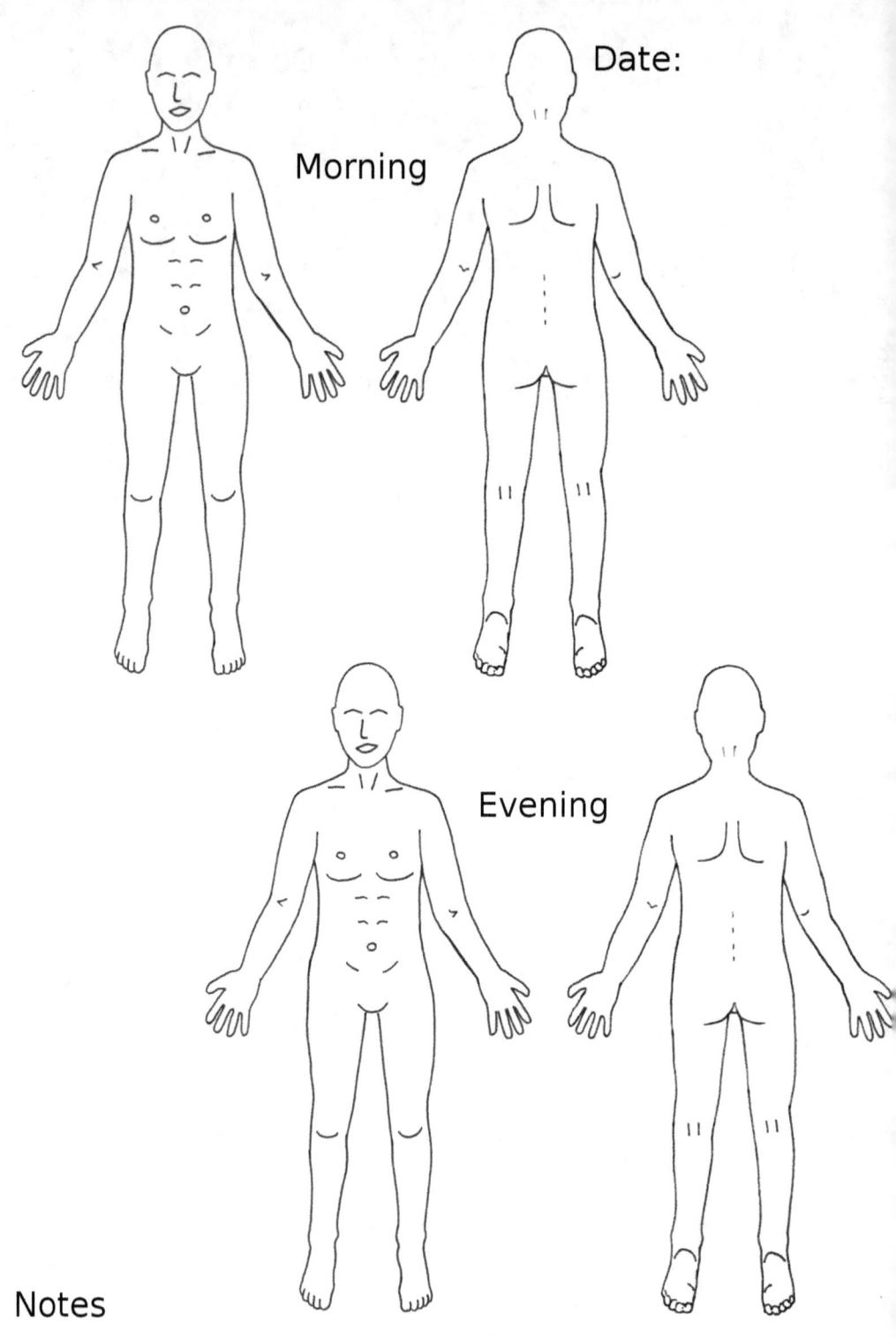

Date:

Morning

Evening

Notes

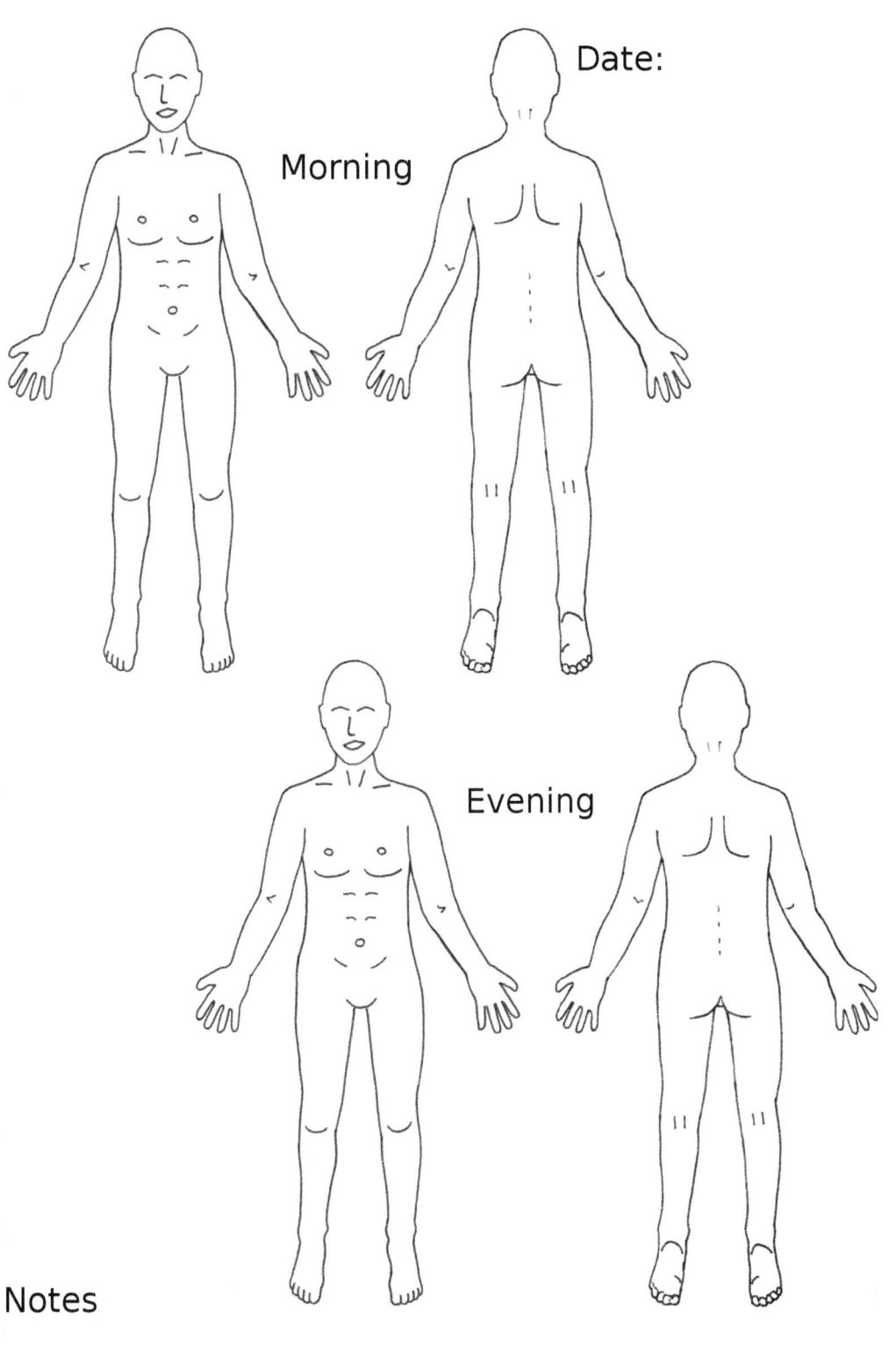

Morning

Date:

Evening

Notes

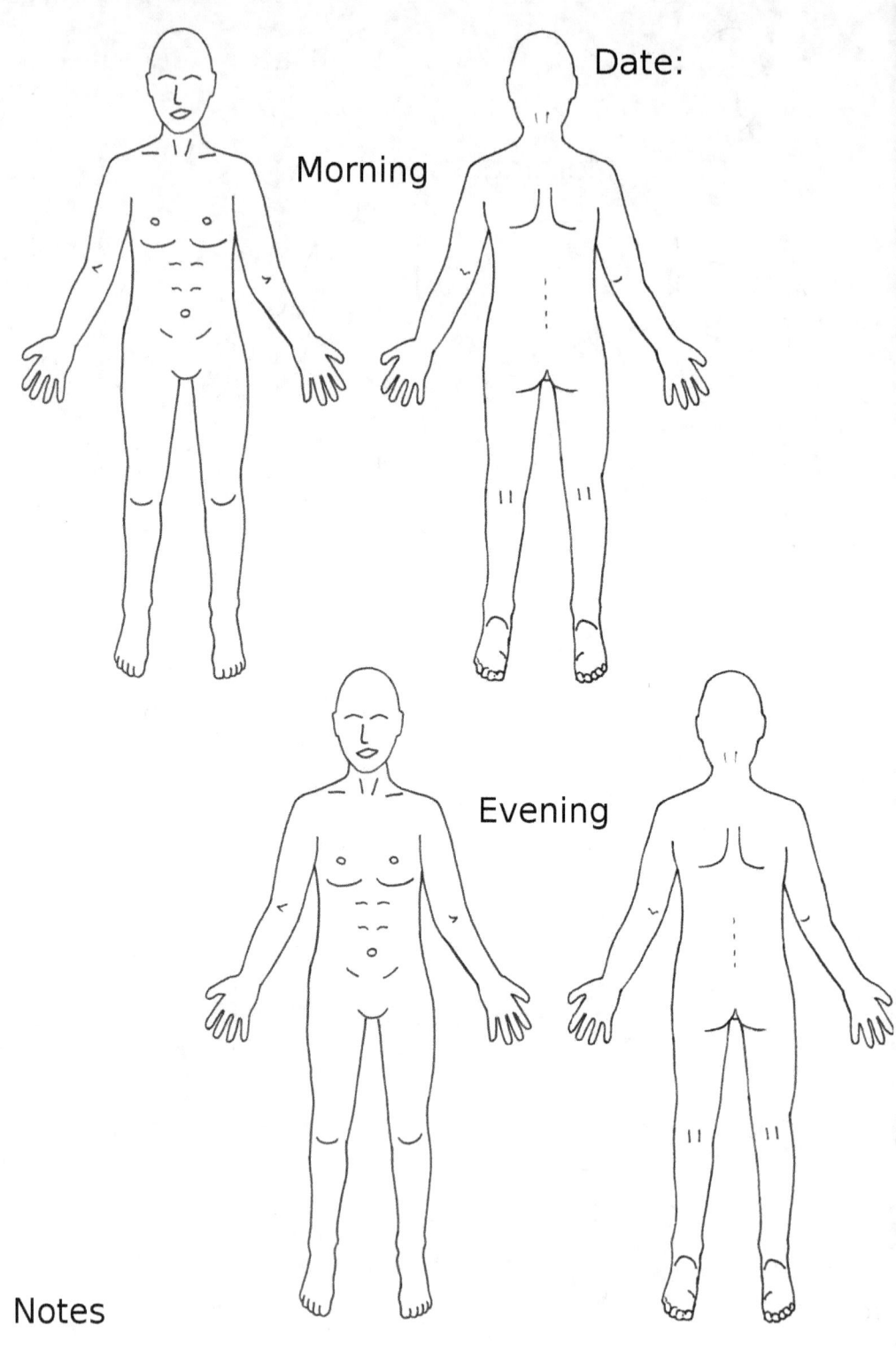

Morning

Date:

Evening

Notes

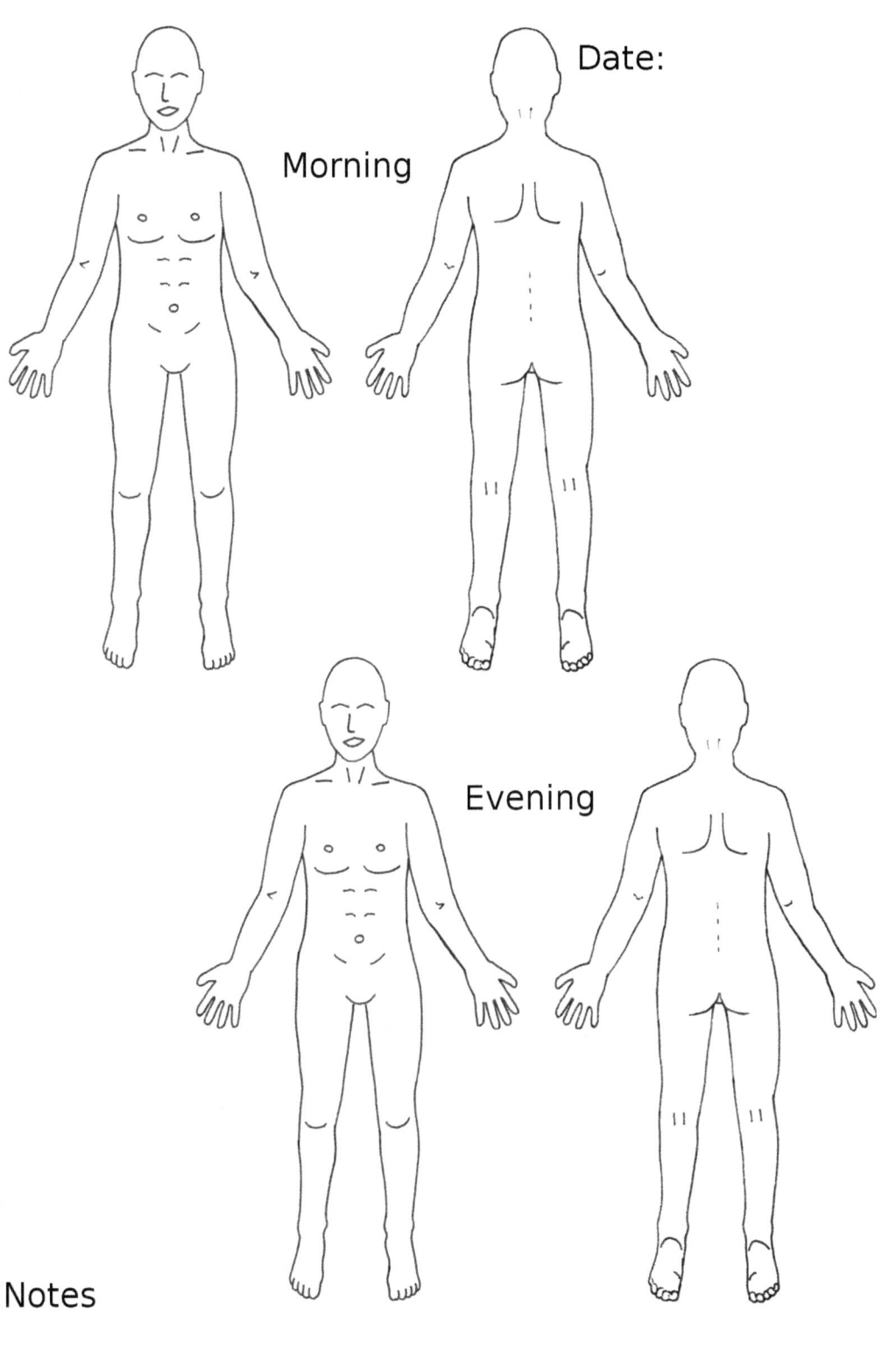

Date:

Morning

Evening

Notes

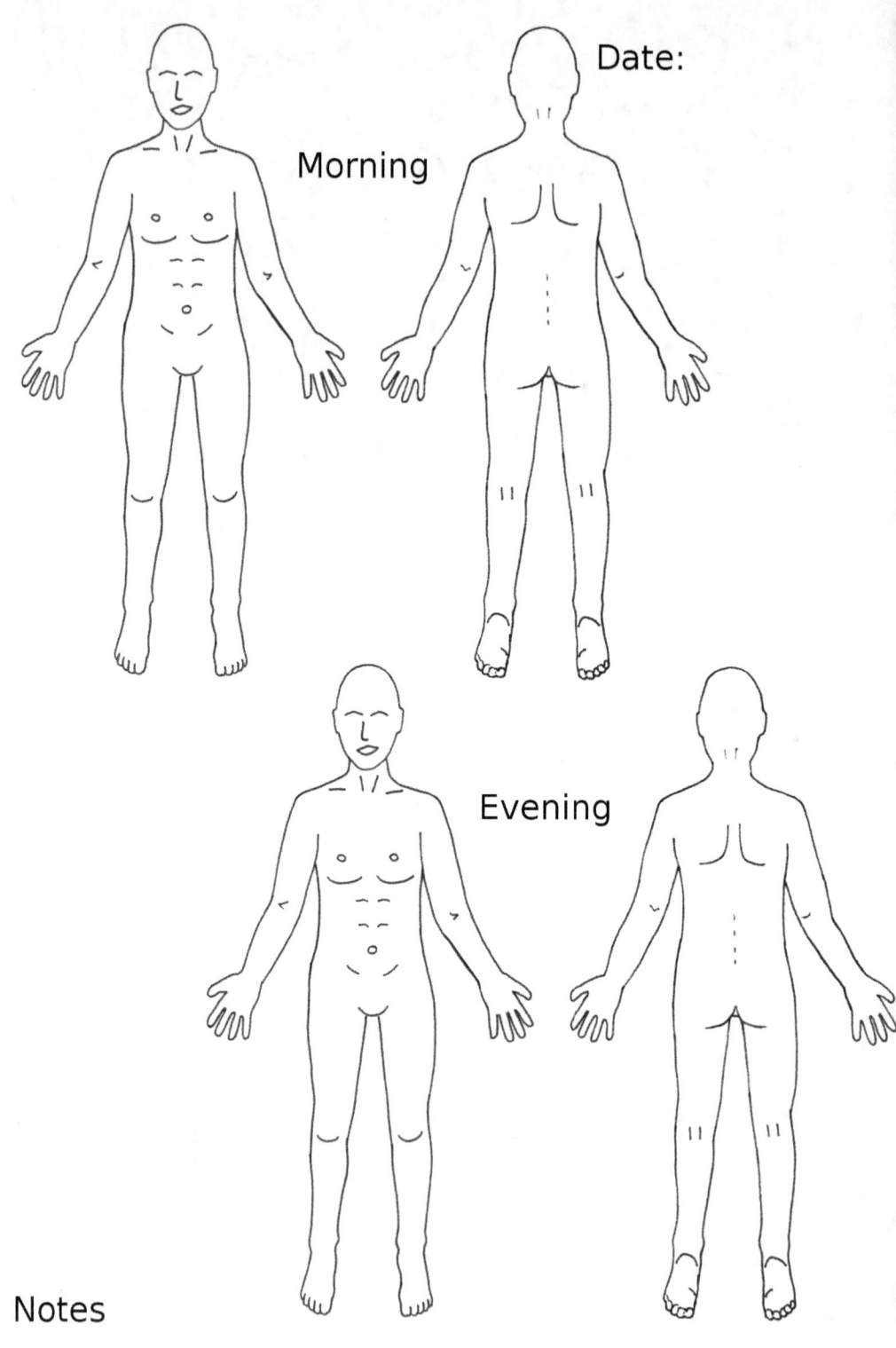

Morning

Date:

Evening

Notes

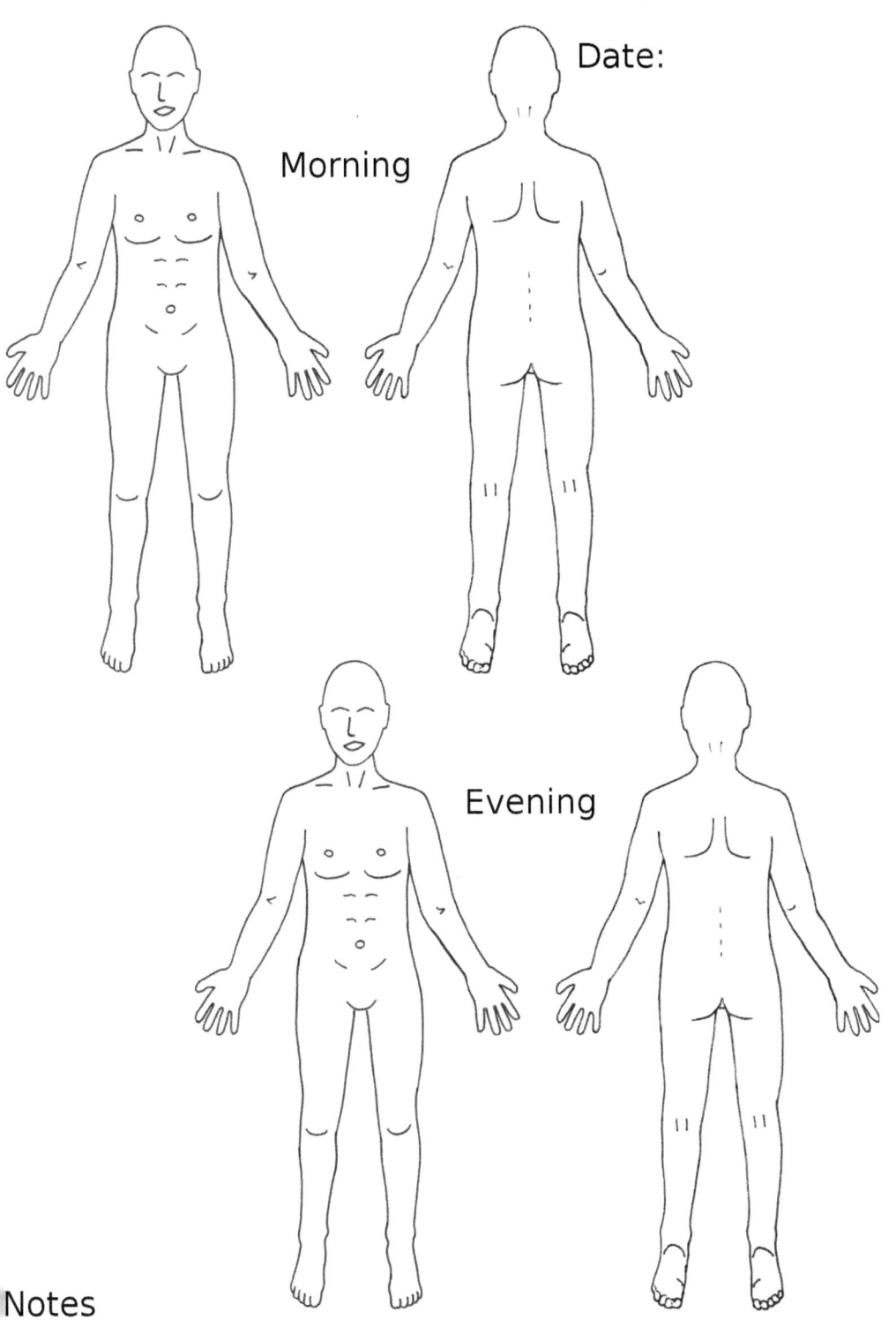

Date:

Morning

Evening

Notes

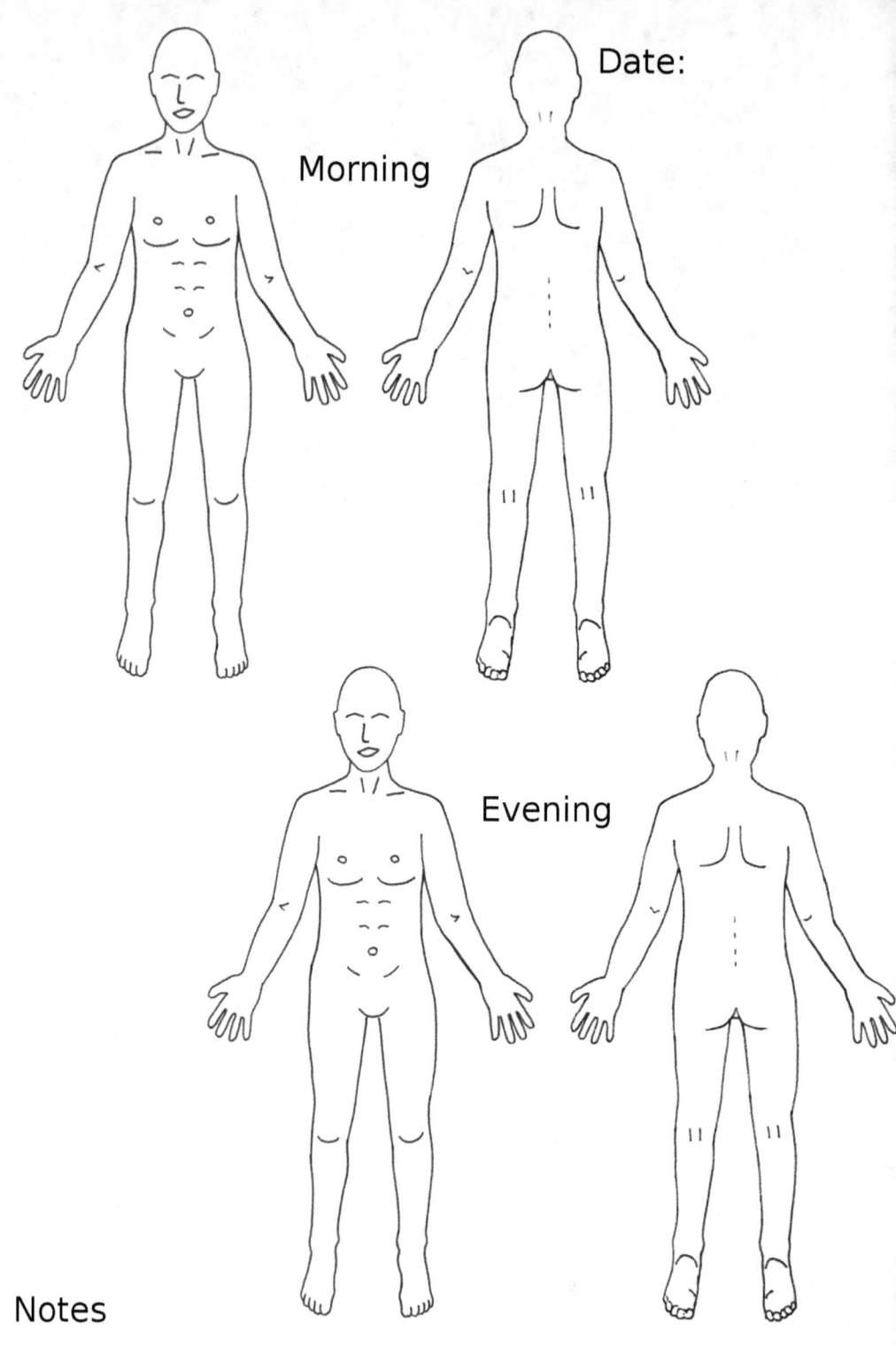

Morning

Date:

Evening

Notes

www.ingramcontent.com/pod-product-compliance
Lightning Source LLC
Chambersburg PA
CBHW060436290526
45791CB00002B/959